"When I read H[...]e good. The bad. [...] is journey. It really helps you realize that, while we all look different, live in different places, and have different life experiences, the human experiences of challenge and triumph is familiar to us all."
*Angela Hayes | Managing Director,*
*Mission Support Communications*
*American Cancer Society*

"I have always said that I am not grateful for having cancer, but I am grateful for the blessings it has brought. Dan is one of those blessings. He has many gifts, especially writing and storytelling. But he, himself, is a gift to everyone who is fortunate enough to know him. Thanks Dan, for all you give unconditionally."
*Teri Griege | Survivor, Triathlete, Founder and CEO*
*Powered By Hope Foundation*

"Dan Duffy has endured struggles that most can't imagine, and not only endured, but has thrived. In this remarkable, emotional, poignant and surprisingly funny book, he shares not only what he learned as he battled cancer, but what it means for all of us in the daily fights of life. There is reason for hope...and you'll know why after you read this book!"
*John O'Leary | International Speaker and Author*

"I thought it was funny and personal and very realistic. That is a good combination given the severity of the topic and circumstances. Well done!"
*Doug Ulman*
*President and CEO, Pelotonia*
*Former President and CEO, LIVESTRONG*

# THE HALF BOOK

*He's taking his ball and going home.*

Dan Duffy

Lucky Bat Books

*A Lucky Bat Book*

*The Half Book: He's Taking His Ball and Going Home
Copyright 2015 by Dan Duffy*

*Cover Artist: Dave Cutler
Cover Design: Brandon Swann*

*Published by Lucky Bat Books
10 9 8 7 6 5 4 3 2 1*

*All rights reserved.*

*No portion of this book may be transmitted or reproduced in any manner, including photocopying, without written permission of the author. For purposes of reviews, short quotations may be reproduced without prior permission.*

*This book also available in digital formats.*

# Contents

To Whom I'm Grateful—vii
A Not-Sappy Foreword—xi
Prologue: Enough—xv

**1**
The Twinge—1

**2**
Halloween—11

**3**
Change of Plans—25

**4**
Doesn't Ever Leave the Airport—35

**5**
The Red Herrings—45

**6**
The Tip of My Iceberg—57

**7**
Three Little Words—67

**8**
Four Little Words—73

**9**
My Second Great Embarrassment—85

**10**
Dodged the Bullet (I Thought)—91

## CONTENTS

**11**
May or May Not Cause Bone Pain—99

**12**
Hold Me—107

**13**
The Beauty of Week Three—119

**14**
Call Me Douchemael—125

**15**
The Elephant—133

**16**
My Bucket of Suck—139

**17**
Going Home—147

**18**
The Celebration of Life—157

**19**
Bartender! One More Round!—169

**20**
The PET Scan—177

**21**
Pulling a Jesus—183

**22**
Losing Lefty—191

# CONTENTS

**23**
The Miracles—197

**24**
It Can't Be Done—205

**25**
Haiti—215

**26**
The Accidental Activist—223

Epilogue:
Your Services are No Longer Required—233

About the Author   237

# TO WHOM I'M GRATEFUL

This book should never have happened. I'm still fairly stunned it's made it this far. My life is an embarrassment of riches, and there are some wonderful people I need to thank.

To my wife Stephanie: you have saved me in every way imaginable. You are my literal everything, and I love you with every fiber of my being.

To my sons Sam and Ben: you will always be my greatest achievement. Your daddy is so proud of the young men you are, and he loves you so much.

To my parents Ray and Marie, and to my brother Gavin: you are a constant reminder that family is everything, and I'm so blessed to have you as my rock. "I love you" is an understatement.

To Michele, Dan, Courtney, Pat, Tiffiny, Jack and Debbie, Jess and Matt: thank you for not being my in-law family, but my family. I love you all!

To Kira, Arden, Gavin, Katie, Hayden and Owen: with you as our future, I have great hope for humanity. Uncle Dan loves you!

To my mentor, Wayne: words can't express the gratitude for all you have meant to me. You and Courtney are friends and models for how humans should treat each other.

To my Half Fund partner, Joe: Thank you for your voice of reason, your tough love, and your friendship. Something tells me a few more dimensions are about to kick in.

To Kelly, Muzzy, and David: Thank you for agreeing to come on this bumpy ride with us from the beginning. Your friendship and ideas have been invaluable. And to Mandi and Linda: You have no idea what you're in for, so buckle up. Thank you for your trust and support. We're in great hands with you.

To Amy: This book doesn't get written without you. Thank you for your passion, your encouragement, your voice, and for the writing mantra, "Butt to seat."

To Courtney, Shane, Cindie, Judith, and everyone at Lucky Bat: Are you sure you want to go through with publishing this? I've never done this before. I mean, I'm so grateful, but it's not too late to back out, because quite frankly, I have no idea what I'm doing.

To Dave. Your art staggers and fractures me.

To Sarah, to April and Angela from the ACS, to Vince from Rabbit Bandini, to Jon, to Kevin and Jen, to Kim from the CSC, to the folks from LIVESTRONG, to Courtney and Steve and D.C., to Margie from FOX 2, to Mark from KMOX, to Angela and the folks from Unidev, to Todd, to Judy and Angela and Jerry and everyone from TEDx Sarasota, to Maneli, to Craig, to Karen, to Dr. Diane Carson, to Pauline from the IAC in New York, and to Megacita: thank you for a life filled with "Cinderella Moments," the kind that Matthew Broderick talked about in *Biloxi Blues* when he said, "…not enough to kill you, but just enough to keep you from walking straight."

To Richard, Chris, Subash, Len, Liz, Otter, Larry, Brian, Butter, Isabel, Beads, Bo, Laura, Louis, Art, Dave, Andy, Robby, Spencer, Mike, Randy, Gary and all the kids at Stepstone, Jake and Todd and Craig and Rick and Josh and the entire Effingham crew, to Shelly and Ed, to Bob, to Bobby and Mick and all of my brothers from De Smet Jesuit, and to everyone who played a part in the lowest point of my life: thank you for making me laugh, for not looking at me differently, and for treating me as normally as you possibly could in the most abnormal of situations. It made a difference then. It still makes one today.

To Seamus, to Yokasta and Timothy, to Liz A, to Sarah, to Alexis, Tayler, and Adam Horwitz, to the amazing Tony D, to Jeremy and the Becky, to Matt, to Amy, to Scott and Lauren and everyone at KolbeCo (especially Lily), to Rick and Donna, to everyone at Funds2Orgs, to Jessica, to Jen and your amazing kiddos, to Fred and Elizabeth, to Colby, to Parker, to Bud, to the folks at McGurk's, to Scott and staff from the former Big Bang, to Jim and John, to DJ and the crazy talent at Coolfire, to Sara, to Ted and Katie, to Joe and everyone at Genovese Jewelers, to Damien and Jen, to Matty Birk, to Carolyn and Ali, to my extended Immac family, to Reginald, to Meg, to Cara and Billy from Hope4YAWC, to Margie from STLMGAC, to Norm, to Glove and Guy and Buzz and Vic and Jen, to Michele, to Suzy, to KC and everyone at the ECMG, to Donny, to Travis, to Lisa, to Christine, to Scotty A, and to all who have helped us to further our mission in different ways: you have kept the stories flowing, you constantly inspire me, and I'm so thankful for you.

To Renata and Kelly and Scott and everyone from the Cancer Support Community, to Shane (formerly with the Huffington Post) and to all who have ever shared our blogs, to Marta from FCCLA, to Adam, to Lisa, to Jeanette from St. Louis Magazine, to Nancy from HEC, and to Matthew and everyone from *Stupid Cancer*: thank you so much for giving us a platform, and trusting us not to mess it up.

To Doctors Burt Needles, Richard Pennell, Leonard Gaum, and Scott Bakunas: thank you for saving my life.

To Kim, to Teri, to Dr. Sheri, to Andy, to Cesar, to Ed, to Katie, to Scott, to Ann, to Jill, to Nick, to Casey, to Donna from *Living Like a Lady*, to Hannah and Caleb, to Rachel, to BJ, and to all of my friends who have battled cancer and who continue to battle: thank you for a never ending supply of hope and courage, even when you don't feel hopeful or courageous.

To the families and friends of Todd, Deb, Leann, Mackenzie, and to all of those I know who have succumbed to this disease: may you feel a semblance of comfort knowing that they will always be there to influence us, and to remind us why we're doing all of this in the first place.

To the memory of my own Pop and my Uncle Declan: cancer took your bodies far too soon.

To you, the reader: thank you for buying this book, thank you for reading it, and if you were to share it, I would thank you for that, too. And if you're reading a stolen copy of this book, please feel free to give it to someone who could use it. No questions asked.

To anyone I may have unintentionally forgotten. I do that sometimes. I'm not proud of it, and I apologize.

And finally, to God: thank you for my life, my near-death experiences, my Bear, my family and friends, my successes and lack thereof, and for cancer. Because without cancer…

…no one is reading this.

You made it to the end of the list! Yay, you! If you're still awake, please turn the page.

# A NOT-SAPPY FOREWORD

by Amy Marxkors

Here's what you need to know about Dan Duffy: he has red hair, he is the reason the Adam's Mark Hotel in downtown St. Louis had to replace the carpet on the 11th floor, and he was banned for life from the Library Limited bookstore in Clayton. That bookstore is now out of business. The Adam's Mark is now a Hyatt. Dan Duffy still has red hair.

Point: Mr. Duffy.

"So, how did you guys meet?"

"Online."

Ours began as a modern friendship. By this, of course, I mean Facebook. Dan reviewed one of my books for *The Huffington Post* and reached out to me regarding a potential editing project. After several flailing attempts to schedule a meeting, we finally convened at Blueprint Coffee on a Friday morning in the middle of December. Little did we know these Friday morning conferences at Blueprint would become ritual or that the editing project (which never happened) would serve simply as the rocket booster to *The Half Book* space shuttle (which didn't yet exist).

*The Half Book*, that is, not the space shuttle.

In retrospect, this book couldn't *not* exist. Dan Duffy was born to tell stories.

If the *I Ching* and *National Enquirer* had a lovechild, that child would be Dan Duffy. His accounts are colorful, vibrant, hopeful, and unfailingly infused with hilarity and unexpected metaphor. But it's not just the way he tells stories: it's the curiosity and joy motivating the narrative.

Dan Duffy finds people fascinating, and that fascination leads to wonder and empathy. It's a quality that's hard to pin down at first, but as you listen to him describe the time he used a sock puppet to harass Ann B. Davis (yes, Alice from *The Brady Bunch*) or the time he and his wife traveled to the Vatican to have their marriage blessed by the pope (he squeezed into a suit tailored for a man thirty-pounds lighter, and she wore her sister's eighth-grade confirmation dress), you realize what makes Dan Duffy so special. He is utterly devoid of apathy and cynicism.

Even after suffering a nasty death threat in the form of cancer, he remains mesmerized by the human experience. Perhaps that's why he spent twenty years telling other peoples' stories in film, television, and radio (winning multiple prestigious awards, I might add) before undertaking the project of his own narrative.

It's also why he and his good friend, Joe Farmer, turned the nonprofit world on its head when they conceived and created The Half Fund as a way to use art to raise cancer awareness and education. The first of its kind, The Half Fund finances films, television shows, books, and music that illustrate the realities of a cancer diagnosis. Even more, half of all the proceeds from those projects goes to the cancer charity of the artist's choice, and the other half is funneled back into The Half Fund to help sponsor more projects. In other words, Dan and Joe concocted a way to channel the power of storytelling into a trident of sorts—a self-regenerating, cancer-fighting, not-for-profit trident.

How cool is that?

Now, I was given strict instruction not to write a sappy foreword, so let me just say that Dan Duffy is one of my favorite humans on this planet, and I am honored to have even the tiniest part in the making of *The Half Book*. I am grateful for his zest (super zest, really) and unremitting enthusiasm for life. I know that everyone who reads *The Half Book* will feel the same way I did each time I left Blueprint Coffee: inspired to make things happen, encouraged to pursue my crazy dreams, and reminded never to let my curiosity fade.

Trust me on this—you will be a better human for knowing Dan Duffy.

Unless, of course, you were ever associated with Library Limited or the Adam's Mark Hotel. In that case, you have my condolences.

Sincerely,

*Amy Marxkors*

# PROLOGUE: ENOUGH

"**W**e've got a problem, sir."

This is not something you want to hear from your pilot.

"What's the problem?"

*God, please don't say we are low on gas or a wing fell off.*

"We've got a pretty massive headwind from that thunderhead. It's taking all I can to get back to the jump run. If I can't get you far enough past the airport, you're gonna end up miles away."

A year earlier, over chicken wings and beer, my friends and I had the brilliant idea to learn how to skydive. Six weeks later, we spent eight hours at Quantum Leap Skydiving Center in Sullivan, Missouri, learning what and what not to do when jumping out of a plane at fourteen thousand feet.

Fourteen. Thousand. Feet.

*Whiskey. Tango. Foxtrot.*

Throughout the class, we learned just how many things could go wrong, and what we needed to do in any situation we may encounter. Always turn at ninety degree angles, and to the left. Breathe. Power lines are not your friends; avoid them. And no matter what, don't let go of the rip chord when you pull. If it ends up in some corn field, you owe the drop zone a case of beer.

*What?*

We also needed to be apprised of what to do in case of an actual emergency. An issue with the main parachute is rare, but we needed to be prepared in case we had to deploy the reserve chute. We repeated the mantra "Look. Reach. Look. Pull. Reach. Pull. Arch. Check Canopy…" approximately fifty times. And then we were made to repeat it fifty times more. They were taking no chances with their new class of students.

Just when our heads could swim no more, it was time to go up. Chris was the first to jump. He was flanked by two jumpmasters—expert skydivers employed not to let us do anything stupid in the air. He jumped, pulled, landed. The moment his feet hit earth, he broke a smile bigger than his face.

"Never doing that shit again!"

Grant was the second jumper.

"Freakin' awesome! Nope!"

My brother, Gavin, was the third. When he touched down, he spewed every expletive in the book…in a good way. He was hooked. He didn't know that he would *unhook* himself after jump number five a few weeks later.

Richard and I were the last to go. In fact, we were the last jumpers of the day, which meant they had enough jumpmasters to permit us to go up in the plane together. His triumvirate jumped out before I did, and it was quite the thing to see. And feel. As the mass of bodies exploded from the back of the plane, the tail kicked sideways. The reality of my situation T-boned my psyche.

*What the hell am I doing?*

We then walked to the back door of the plane, and did what's called a "hotel check." I looked to my right at my first jumpmaster. "Okay?" I asked.

"Okay," she replied. That's checking in. I did the same with the other jumpmaster, who was hanging on to the outside of the plane. That's checking out.

And then in an instant, the exhaust smell, the roar of the engine, and even the plane, itself, seemed to disappear.

*Freefall.*

The jump was a bit blurry at first. The noise was deafening as we fell to the earth at a buck-twenty. Once I regained my bearings, I looked to my right to see my jumpmaster smiling at me. Oddly, her composure relaxed me enough to focus on flying. I looked to the other jumpmaster on my left, who gave me a thumbs-up. I looked at the ground, which wasn't, to my surprise, racing up to crush my body at breakneck speed. We were so high up, it felt more like a gentle fall.

My gaze moved to my altimeter for my mark of 5,500 feet. This was where I would start the process that even professional jumpers employ: Look. Reach. Pull. Arch. Check canopy.

My chute opening was a funny thing. I traveled from 120 miles-per-hour to zero in less than two seconds, which I have to say did a number on my anal cavity. And somewhere in there, I believe I saw the bottom of my own feet.

The sheer violence of the wind gave way to a beautiful, eerie silence. After a few seconds to process all was happening, the serenity was broken by Jim's voice through the one-way speaker on my chest strap as he talked me all the way down.

"Turn a little left. Don't cross the runway. Doing amazing, man. You've got this!"

I loved it. I laughed. I may have shed a tear, though it was probably just ragweed, or possibly the result of the minute-long 120 miles-per-hour breeze on my contact lenses. As I landed and I saw Richard's face a moment later, it was like I was looking in a mirror. We both knew that we were going to take this all the way.

Just a short year later, almost to the day, I would lament my own stupidity for taking this all the way.

The day started innocently enough. It was a Friday afternoon, and the drop zone was open for some happy hour jumps. The sky was gloriously blue as I drove the hour from my house. If I was lucky, I might get two or three jumps in before meeting my friends for dinner that evening.

Mother Nature had other ideas. A paltry five minutes before my first jump, a thunderhead bore down and walloped the drop zone, dumping an unimaginable amount of rain and hail across the metal roof of the battened-down airplane hangar.

The building was thrashed for a solid fifteen minutes. And then all was quiet. We opened the hangar door to reveal that glorious blue sky, part deux. The thunderhead was three miles east of the airport. We mocked it. *That's all you've got?*

No, actually.

"Define miles away," I said to the pilot. I hoped he didn't notice the reticence in my voice or the swamp accumulating in my shorts.

"Like…literally miles away," said the pilot. "We should probably land."

"Dude, I've got this," I said with all the false-bravado of someone who had twenty-four jumps under his belt.

"You sure?" he asked.

"I'm sure," I lied.

T'was not my smartest decision.

As soon as I jumped, I knew something was wrong. Flipping wildly was my first clue. It took every bit of my basic skill to stop pulling my mid-air Greg Louganis. Once I stabilized and found a column of air on which to fall, I searched for the airport.

*Airport? Here, airport! Come to daddy! Where the hell is the stupid airport? Why the hell didn't the stupid pilot land?* Oh, yeah, that's right, because I asked him not to.

I looked down. No airport. I looked up at the horizon. I turned ninety degrees to the right. Ninety more. *Wait, is that…the airport? Yes!* It was miles…and miles…and miles away. *Shit.*

One of the first things we learned in our skydiving curriculum was how to track. Instead of having your arms out in front of you and your knees bent, you pull your arms back to your sides and straighten your legs. On the surface, that may sound like you would fly into the earth like a dart. In reality, it propels you forward in more of a straight line.

The one thing the instructors tell you never to do, however, is track parallel to the runway. They drop you parallel to the runway; tracking in the same direction increases the risk of colliding with another jumper, which is a very bad thing for many reasons, not the least of which is getting knocked out before you have a chance to deploy your parachute.

The word "impact" is the actual cause-of-death term used for someone who dies from a chute not opening.

*Impact.* It even sounds painful.

But this situation was different. I threw the no-parallel-tracking rule out the window. My goal was to get back to the airport, and by God, I was going to do it. I pulled my arms back and straightened my legs, effectively turning myself into a human javelin. I felt the wind trying to hold me back, but I was having none of it.

I made a tremendous amount of headway. I had only been tracking for about a minute, but the airport was now in reach. At about three thousand feet, well below my comfort level, I finally pulled my pilot chute, which was attached to my parachute. It caught the air, violently ripping the main canopy out of my container.

As the canopy fully opened, I looked down. I was less than a mile away from the target. My gamble had paid off. I would make it back to the airport.

*Not so fast,* said the wind. *Don't you know anything about the laws of aerodynamics?*

Whether you are under canopy, soaring in a glider, or landing an Airbus A-380, the laws of aerodynamics don't change. You fly into the wind if you have the wind to fly into. It helps to slow you down. It's your friend.

Now while I don't know the intricacies of the other modes of aeronautical transport, I do know that while under canopy, on a dead-calm day, my speed was roughly twenty miles-per-hour. The wind decided to have a little fun with me. It battered my face and buffeted my chest at about twenty-two miles-per-hour. In other words, I was descending slightly *backwards*, away from the airport.

*How do experienced skydivers create speed?* My inexperienced mind raced for a solution. *Think!*

And then it hit me: they swoop. A parachute rig has two brake lines that allow you to steer by pulling on one side or the other. When you pull both, you slow down. While experienced jumpers use the lines to finesse a landing, they use the actual riser straps attached to the canopy to steer. These straps produce a more violent turn, but they can generate a ton of speed if you do it right.

I had seen it countless times, but I'd never actually done it, partially from fear, and partially because I was so inexperienced. Newbie jumpers were forbidden to even try it at Quantum Leap.

Of course, I had already broken several rules that day. What was one more? I pulled on my right riser strap. Nothing happened. I pulled a little harder. I barely moved. I yanked it down.

*Motherfletcher!*

I raced to the right at a speed for which I was not quite prepared. I let go of the right riser and yanked on the left.

*Whoosh!*

My parachute kicked hard from right to left, and for a brief moment, it felt as if my feet were higher than the canopy. I immediately let go of the left riser, too scared to move.

*H…ho…holy…holy shit! Never doing that again! Never-never-never!*

On the plus side, I had generated enough speed to cut through the wind, albeit briefly. I was at the edge of the drop zone now, slowly moving forward, and about four hundred feet off the ground. The adrenaline was pumping through my body like I had never known. It became intoxicating.

And then, in an unexpected way, my utter terror melded into sheer balls in my newfound ability. I had just pulled off a textbook swoop.

*I have totally got this.*

I didn't have this.

Dealing with headwind is one thing. Dueling a crosswind is quite another. One blew in from my right, swinging me to the left. As I wrestled to control my new pendulum predicament, I looked down to see that I was about sixty feet from landing on top of the airplane hangar.

*Are you kidding me?*

I was pissed.

I grabbed my right brake line and pulled down hard, sending me away from the building.

I released the right and pulled down hard on the left.

I repeated this over and over and over until I was twenty feet off the ground.

Finally, I let go of both brake lines and wailed like a jockey with a hemorrhoid flare-up. Everyone at the drop zone stopped to look at the foaming-at-the-mouth screaming lunatic gently lowering down to the ground.

I could barely feel my foot touch the earth. It was the gentlest landing I had ever pulled off. Jim, a man who teaches Navy Seals how to jump, applauded. I had never worked so hard for anything in my life.

Ever.

I knelt down before I fell down and I touched the grass with my hands, not quite believing what had just happened. I don't really know how close I actually came, but I felt that I had somehow cheated death. I looked up to God and thanked him for sparing me for the third time.

---

I thought about that day as I looked up at the water-stained drop ceiling while sitting in the most uncomfortable, chartreuse, genuine pho-naugahyde recliner ever conceived by man or ape. I asked God how many more times he would let me cheat death as the poisonous chemotherapy slowly dripped into my bloodstream.

# THE
# HALF
# BOOK

# 1

## THE TWINGE

"We ready to go, Danny?"
"Yep, we're set."
"You feel good about it?"
"I do."
"I like you, Dan."
"I like you too, Steve."
"No, I really like you…"
Punch.

Steve is truly one of the funniest, most intelligent people I've ever met. In the summer of 2001, he was one half of the nationally syndicated Steve and DC radio show. It was the last Friday in May, and we were readying his home for one our biggest shows of the year, the annual "Summer Kick-Off Pool Party from Steve's House" broadcast. We had a hell of a time getting the name on the bumper sticker.

When I look back today, I'm still amazed at how we even came together in the first place. It was a mixture of divine providence, hard work, perseverance, and dumb luck.

Steve and DC came to St. Louis in 1991 by way of Alabama and New Orleans. They were irreverent, funny, and controversial. Like any great stalker, I was their number one fan.

I first heard Steve and DC after I had escaped high school. At that point in my life, I was unprepared, or rather, unwilling to give higher education the ol' college try. I worked for a year as a courier driver while taking a few culinary courses to see if I wanted to become a chef. I quickly realized that cooking was not my life's work.

"What do you mean I'll have to work weekends?"

It wasn't all a waste, though. I learned some rudimentary ice carving (turned a large block into a smaller block) and I learned how to decorate a birthday cake (I defy you to pull off a better icing rose than mine). Oh, and do you know what they call the instrument on which to fashion a rose using a pastry bag full of icing?

It's a rose nail.

I also learned a mantra that I carry with me today: when cooking for guests, if it blows, there's Domino's.

With a career in the culinary industry out of the question, I focused on my delivery boy status until I could figure out something else. And to be honest, I wasn't all that worried at first. I was having a great time doing what I was doing.

# 1: THE TWINGE

My introduction to Steve and DC happened in the car, where I spent every morning driving packages from place to place. I was the perfect captive audience member. And like every great relationship, ours featured a rocky start. When I first heard those two, I thought they sucked. They'd end every phone call with "Love ya!" in perfect two-part harmony. It was truly annoying.

So I'd flip from station to station, or play my A Show of Hands cassette by Rush, but something kept calling me back to listen to Steve and DC, and they grew on me like toenail fungus or a wart...the kind that starts small, almost innocuous, but eventually turns into Whoville.

The kind that requires a prescription for a salve with enough side effects to choke a Clydesdale riding a hippo through a minefield.

The kind that makes the cocktail of leprosy, pinkeye, and gout look like a hangnail.

After a few weeks, they became "appointment radio." I would sit in my car and hold up a package delivery if they were in the middle of something hilarious. Whenever I had to get out, I would try to break "quickest delivery" records just to get back into my car so I wouldn't miss anything.

Double parking. Forgetting to take the keys out of the ignition...or to even turn off the car, for that matter. Bypassing the elevator with extreme prejudice. Airmailing anything that wasn't marked "Fragile." Ignoring the wicked-hot receptionist. Sorry, honey. I've got a date with two guys.

*Did I say that out loud?*

After a year, listening had become an addiction, and the withdrawals at 10:15 a.m. weren't much fun. The pain would double during the rest of the day as I dwelled on the uncertainty that was the rest of my life. My job was supposed to be temporary. Now it was looking like a career. I didn't know what to do. Slowly, my worry gave way to panic.

It was at these low points in my life that God would gently bury His foot in my bum and kick me out of complacency. I truly believe He was responsible for the fifty people who unwittingly got together and gang-banged an epiphany straight into my heart.

I was at a stoplight in downtown St. Louis. The sun was shining, my left arm was tan from continually hanging out of my open window, and there was a slight breeze from the northwest blowing in at five miles per hour. The dew point was fairly low (to the best of my recollection). It was lunchtime, and all the downtown office workers were making their daily pilgrimage to Mecca, otherwise known as T.G.I. Fridays.

*I bet they order potato skins*, I thought. *Fridays invented potato skins. I heart their potato skins. If I were on my way to potato skins right now, I'd have a smile on my face.*

But on this beautiful day, at this beautiful moment, as these fifty business professionals in their business-professional outfits walked past my car, I stopped looking at their wingtips and looked up at their faces.

Not one of them was smiling. Not. One.

After I completed my next delivery, I radioed our base, telling them that I was going to be out of the car for a half-hour lunch. Only, I never left my car. I sat in the driver's seat, radio off, and tried to rationalize what I had just witnessed.

I reasoned that I spent the majority of my waking life making deliveries in my car. I reasoned further that it was more than likely that most people spend the majority of their waking lives doing what they do for a living. It didn't make sense to me that anyone would choose a career in which he or she would be miserable. It just didn't.

I called our base again, this time to inform them I had eaten a bad batch of potato skins and would be spending the remainder of my afternoon on the toilet. They bought it…no questions asked. And let's face it, bowel issues are like opinions: everyone has them, but no one wants to hear about them.

In reality, I raced home. No cars were in the driveway. (I lived with my parents at the time.) This was good. I wanted to be alone with my thoughts and plans. I went to my room, closed the door, and grabbed a pen and notepad from the shelf of my gargantuan 1980's headboard with cabinets and mirrors and a disco ball.

I spent the next hour writing down every single thing that I'd ever wanted to do in my life. The list was surprisingly long and ranged from game show host to priest.

The first career paths whittled away were anything illegal or somehow related to porn. Next to die where the occupations that required more than two years of college. Sorry, psychiatry. Sorry, priesthood.

The whittling continued and continued and continued, until finally I was left with one option.

*Steve and DC.*

For several minutes, I tried to talk myself out of it. But my mind was smiling—perma-grin smiling—and I knew I was about to make the rightest decision of my life.

St. Louis has a school called Broadcast Center, where the instructors are actual working professionals who teach nothing but how to work at a radio station. The curriculum consists of commercial production, sales and marketing, and announcing. The instructors teach every broadcasting basic that exists, help you polish your skills, and then shove you out of the nest and into the world.

Our placement director was a man who is famous in his own right. A St. Louis native, he has appeared in some very, very large films. At the beginning of *Ocean's Eleven* (the one with George Clooney and Brad Pitt), there's a scene where Livingston Dell (played by Eddie Jemison) tells the FBI agent, "Don't, don't, don't, don't touch that." The next line is, "Hey, Radio Shack. Relax." That was our placement director.

As I was getting close to graduation, he called me into his office.

"How'd you like to start your career in Sioux Falls, South Dakota?"

I politely declined. He took this two ways: beggars can't be choosers, and this kid has moxie.

His next visit didn't go quite so well.

"How about Cape Girardeau?"

At least this one was in my home state. "What's the job?"

"Ten to six, board-opping for minimum," he said, smiling. He shouldn't have been smiling; this is a job you wouldn't wish on your mother-in-law. "Board-opping" translated to pushing buttons for eight hours during the graveyard shift for less than $4.50 an hour. I told him I wasn't interested. He cursed under his breath as he walked out of the room.

I do think he was trying to look out for me, but I wasn't prepared to settle. I knew I didn't have the chops to work mornings or afternoons—when the big boys play—but I also didn't want to end up doing something that would make me miss courier driving. Plus, I was afraid that if I took the first job that came along, I'd be pigeon-holed as "the guy who's crazy talented at button pushing" or become so miserable in my first radio gig that I'd quit without trying to find the next step.

I put everything I have into everything I do. I'm not into baby steps.

So two days later, when I thought enough time had passed that he wouldn't kill me, I walked into his office to ask for his help.

"I'd like to work for Steve and DC."

"I can't get you a job there, Dan. You have no experience."

"Well, can you at least help me get an internship?"

"Dan, they have two interns. They don't need a third."

I thanked him for his lack of help and walked out. This was one of the last times we ever talked.

The betrayal I felt while sitting on my bed later that day consumed my soul. *How dare that effer?. He just wants to pad the score so he can say that everyone who goes to his school gets a job in radio!* I was going for the throat and making mincemeat out of him. Silently. To myself.

And out of my anger came my solution: *Hell, I should get my own internship there!*

I grabbed a pen and sheet of paper and did what, at the time, was the only way to communicate with someone before the days of Twitter and Facebook and universal email: I wrote them a letter.

I don't remember the exact contents of the letter, but I know I tried to make it funny, playful, and completely serious in my effort to secure an internship. I also wrote something along the lines of, "I know you have two interns, and I'm not trying to take either of their places. All I want is a chance." This was a Tuesday.

I brought the letter to the radio station and left it at the front desk with the receptionist. This was a Wednesday.

My brother knocked on my bedroom door. "Dan, there's some DC guy on the phone for you." This was a Friday.

"Hello?"

"Dan, it's DC from Steve and DC. How are you?"

"Holy shit! Really?"

DC laughed. "Yeah, really. Our producer, Courtney, read your letter. She gave it to Steve and I, and we want to have you in for an interview. Are you interested?"

"Absolutely!" (I wanted to say, "Whose dick to I have to suck to get to do this?" but I refrained.)

Three days later, on a Monday morning after the show, I met Steve, DC, and Kim, their newsperson. I was on such a high; I remember almost nothing about the meeting. I do remember walking out of the building, looking up, and simply saying, "Please."

An hour later, Kim called me with the good news. They wanted me to help her gather news stories, traffic reports, weather, and other sundry items. It was the greatest day of my life. As I drove to Broadcast Center that day, I thought about everything I would say to the placement director, about how I got my foot in the door without his help and how I resented him for not helping me.

But as I got closer to the school, I realized I wouldn't say anything at all. Things happened the way they were supposed to. I finally found something in my life I had to fight for, and I had to rely on my own character choices to make it happen. I jumped into the deep end, and once I hit the water, I threw off the safety of my water wings and swam like my life depended on it.

―

# 1: THE TWINGE

Seven years later, at the annual "Summer Kick-Off Pool Party from Steve's House" broadcast, we would all be swimming in the morning, live on the air. We had worked hard to get the broadcast gear ready for the show. All I had to do was grab the last few cables off the floor and haul them—along with one last beer—to our engineer, Sam.

I searched the living room until I found the cables buried under a mound of couch pillows. I leaned down to push the cushions out of the way.

And I dropped like a stone.

My lower back seized, and I lost all movement in my right leg, which was holding all of my body weight. I collapsed to my knees and put my hands out to stop myself from face-planting on the carpet. My eyes watered as pain seared my entire being.

Two seconds later, it was gone. As quickly as I had crumpled, the pain disappeared. I was terrified. For the first time in my life, I didn't trust the most basic movements. I grabbed the side of the couch and pulled myself up as slowly as possible. I was afraid the pain would return.

It didn't.

"Dan! Get in here!"

Steve was getting impatient from the other room. Twenty people, a deck of cards, and more beer than *Oktoberfest* awaited my presence. Who was I to hold things up?

# 2

## HALLOWEEN

"For God's sake, make it stop!"
*Click.*
"Fifth one tonight!"

Rob, our head production guy on *Steve and DC*, busted his buttons with pride. It was 12:07 a.m. on October 31, 2001, the night of the annual Halloween show. Each year on Halloween, we would broadcast from the residence of a listener who lived in a possessed, ghost-ridden house. Occasionally, the listener was able to dupe us into thinking that something evil was happening; in reality, they just wanted the bragging rights of hosting the show.

This one, however, was different. Even the lead-up to the show was different. The young mom who lived in the house told us she wanted us there. She also told us she didn't want us there. We never knew which reaction we would get from her on any given day. It was a lesson in patience and persistence.

We got a much better idea of her psyche when Jim, our producer, paid a visit to the house. His report was fairly succinct: "That place is fucked up," prompting a genuine apprehension from almost every cast member.

It was left to the audio production crew (Rob and me) to set the stage. Together, we concocted an intro that was supposed to promote a sense of unease in the listening audience, like the ominous nature of the low, brooding E-F-E chord in the *Jaws* theme.

We scared the living dump out of everyone. Eight minutes of pure hell, starting with a song called *Fritter* by the band Skinny Puppy. It is one of the most frightening pieces of music I've ever heard, and the first time I found it, I said, "This is going in." By the time the intro ended and we went live to the guys, ten people had called to complain that they were having heart palpitations.

Mission accomplished.

And the house…*something* was going on in that house. From the moment I walked through the front door, I was exhausted. I could barely keep my eyes open. And the man who lived there kept trying to kick us out. He was very subtle about it, almost smiling. It was creepy beyond words. The later the show went, the more manic he became. He laughed as we signed off and packed up our gear.

The guilt I felt when I walked out of the house at 2:22 a.m. was soul crushing. I had to get back to the station to help Rob put the re-broadcast together. As I left, the wife of the creepy man looked at me with a look I'll never forget. It was desperate.

## 2: HALLOWEEN

It cried, "Help me." She didn't utter a word. I know DC stayed longer to talk with them, but he wouldn't discuss it with us. I never did hear about the fallout of that night, and it haunts me.

By the end of the regular show that morning, I had been awake since 3:00 a.m. the day before. My brain felt like the floor of a movie theater—after the dollar-show screening of a *Shrek* double feature. Work ended at 11:00 a.m. Everyone on the show left the station with the intention of sleeping for the next sixteen hours.

My phone rang as I opened my car door in the parking lot. It was Richard. We'd been friends since we were fifteen.

"Hello?"

"Ass-cake."

"Hi, Richard."

"Can we use your truck to cart Lombardo's to Union Plaza?"

Richard worked for a pharmacy just two minutes from the radio station. The owners of the pharmacy, Len and one-time-skydiver Grant, were treating everyone to a catered meal of Lombardo's Trattoria, and they asked Richard to pick up the feast, which is no small task in an MG. He wanted to use my Durango. Of course, my brain was tapioca. At that point, I would have said yes if he had asked for my pancreas.

"Be there in three."

I pulled up to the pharmacy, and Richard slid into the passenger seat. From the moment we rolled out of the parking lot, he gave me the third degree about the Halloween show. What was real? What was fake? What *really* happened? Thankfully, Lombardo's was two minutes away, so my release from the Spanish Inquisition came quickly.

Ten minutes later, I carried platters of toasted ravioli into the pharmacy. I was like Baby carrying the watermelon into a dirty dancers' party. And as I rounded the corner, I saw her.

Stephanie.

She had red hair, blue eyes, porcelain skin, a perfect nose, and a smile that arrested me like the time I forgot to pay a speeding ticket that ended up in a bench warrant. My heart skipped several beats, which may or may not have been exacerbated by my complete lack of sleep. She looked over, smiled, and gave me a tiny wave.

It stunned me. Was she even real? The whole thing felt like an out-of-body experience.

*Did that really just happen?* I thought as I continued walking. *Did I see what I think I saw? Was she waving at someone behind me? How long have I been awake?*

I chalked it up to delirium as I made my way back to Grant's office to grab a bite. After I finished a plate of toasted ravioli and flash-fried spinach, I bid my friends goodbye. Before I left, I blurted out, "You know, that Stephanie is really cute in an unattainable sort of way."

"What do you mean unattainable?" Richard asked.

"Because she knows you're my best friend, and that's gotta be strikes one, two, and three against me."

I drove home on autopilot, stripped to my boxers, and passed out.

———

My cell phone would not shut up. It rang for the third time. I looked at the clock on my nightstand. 8:04 p.m. I'd been sleeping for seven hours, and I was not ready to wake up. Fed up, I grabbed the phone.

"What!"

"Dude, get down here." Richard was sauced.

"Where?"

"Schneithorst's." This was our local hangout, owned by the family of our mutual friend, Chris.

"Richard, I'm going back to bed."

"No! Wait! Bad idea. The red head is down here. She's into you."

*Shut the front door.*

"And I suggest if you have to shower, do the French pits-and-ass thing." And then he hung up.

I took the fastest shower of my life, threw on black jeans and a blue shirt, and raced to the bar faster than a rabbit on Cialis. As soon as I walked in, I saw that I was going to be the designated driver for the night. Richard was there, finishing a shot with his girlfriend *du jour*. And Stephanie.

It was pointless for me to try to catch up to three people who'd had a two-hour head start drinking. I ordered a beer at the bar. Ten seconds after my first sip, I was informed that we were leaving Schneithorst's and heading down to a bar in the city called Nadine's. That one sip of beer cost me eight bucks with a tip.

But I got to hang with Stephanie.

The four of us piled into my truck and headed east to downtown St. Louis. Stephanie and I became fast friends in the car. We never stopped talking during the entire twenty-minute ride. She told me about her family and about work. I told her about nothing of any consequence. A friend once counseled me before a blind date: "Never talk about yourself. Keep talking about her. She'll like that." The blind date went horribly, but the advice seemed to be working tonight.

During the one brief lull in the conversation, I turned my head around to ask Richard if he knew how to get to the bar. It was at that moment that I got a view of his girlfriend's bare breasts. He was going to town on her right nipple like a starving baby. I giggled. Stephanie looked at me and then turned to catch Richard playing "Motorboat." She whipped her head forward, throwing her hands to her eyes.

"Oh, my God." She was half-disgusted, half-laughing.

*She has morals and a sense of humor. Bonus.*

Nadine's is an old-fashioned bar in a little hamlet called Soulard, which happens to host the second-largest Mardi Gras party in the United States behind New Orleans. Depending on where you are in Soulard, you'll find yourself in either an oasis of cool or the seventh bowel of hell. Nadine's was on the oasis end, with a really nice outside seating area complete with a full bar and fire pit.

Within minutes of arriving, Stephanie and I realized that we were sitting at the fire pit, alone. Richard had bought each of us a beer, and then he and his girlfriend disappeared.

Stephanie and I continued to get to know each other. Before long, she said, "I'm glad you came out, but I was worried."

"Why?" I asked.

"Because I've had a crush on you for a while."

Every cell in my body blushed. My heart stopped, exploded, and then started beating again, most likely at a lethal rate. I could almost hear the surge of adrenaline coursing through my body.

"Just…wow. I never thought you'd give me a second look. I thought you were so pretty the moment I saw you."

## 2: HALLOWEEN

Where the hell did that come from? I sounded like a *Between You and Me* Hallmark card, and it was pouring out of me. She smiled and blushed and crinkled up her nose. I instantly fell in love.

And this was not a good thing. I had plans that were over two years in the making, and just a few months from now, I planned on them coming to fruition halfway across the country.

I was actually on my second stint with *Steve and DC*. My first ended in May of 1999, when I took a little hiatus to attend the Vancouver Film School. From the time I was a kid, I always wanted to make movies. However, this was destined to be yet another unrequited dream. Back when I made my list of what I wanted to do for a living, filmmaking was not even on the radar. Film school meant a four-year degree (not up for it) and living in California (not moving).

Radio, for the win.

After a few years of waking up at 3:30 every morning, it became less and less fun. The work became less satisfying. My brand of humor with the guys started veering into the mean side, because it was the path of least resistance. Steve would say something, I would make fun of him for his accent or his waistline, everyone in the room would laugh, and we'd break for commercial. It was unchallenging, lowest common denominator radio. I didn't like the person I was becoming, and I was burned out.

This was not lost on my parents, who upon taking me to lunch on St. Patrick's Day of 1998, said, "You're not happy are you?"

"Of course I'm happy," I snapped.

"No you're not," said my mother. "We can hear it in your voice on the air."

"Really?" I asked.

"If you wanted to get out of there, what would you want to do?" my dad asked.

"I'd want to make movies," I said. *Where the hell did that come from?* After what didn't take too much convincing, I made the decision to take some classes at Meramec, the community college in town. It was there that I met Diane, the woman who would teach me more about the pure art of storytelling than anyone before or since. She convinced me to take her advanced class next semester, and then go to a real film school, as she felt this was my calling in life.

It's amazing how things change when someone you respect believes in you, especially someone in the role you want to eventually inhabit. Steve and DC gave me the courage to make a career out of radio, and now Diane gave me the courage to leave everything safe and do something I had never envisioned: pull off an entire career change. It was now or never, as it would just get harder as I got older.

I made the decision to leave before I got too old, too scared, or too jaded to follow a dream. In fact, when I left for Canada, I hadn't planned on coming back to St. Louis. The film school was only a year long, and after graduation, I would either stay in Vancouver, or head down to Hollywood.

But life has a funny way of dropping you exactly where you need to be, especially when you least expect it.

My sole job offer upon graduating film school? A small production house in St. Louis, Missouri. I mean, what are the chances? Slim to none. That's what the chances are.

And when I sent an e-mail to all of my friends letting them know I was coming home for a while, the first person to respond was Steve.

"How'd you like to come back, Danny?" he said in his thick Alabama drawl over a telephone call on my second day home. "We'll even pay you more than you were making, and you can be off whenever you need to shoot." What has two thumbs and couldn't turn it down? This guy! I rationalized that this must be part of a bigger plan. I figured after a year back in my hometown to hone my skills, I would take the next step and move to Hollywood. I had some friends who worked in the industry and were willing to go to bat for me, as were some of my former instructors from film school.

My homecoming was just over a year prior to this moment at Nadine's. In three short months, I would leave St. Louis forever. Yet here I was, falling in love, and there was nothing I could do about it.

After our school-kid-crush sentiments, we stopped talking and just looked at each other. The silence was deafening. Our gaze did not waver. We stared and smiled and didn't think to ask, "What?" I was admiring a piece of God's perfect art, and I couldn't avert my eyes.

But Richard could.

"Assholes, we're going to Attitudes."

"You mean...*Attitudes*, Attitudes?"

"Yep."

Attitudes is a lesbian bar. Richard's girlfriend was thinking of becoming a switch-hitter, and he was going to try to walk himself into a three-way. I kinda wanted to see if he could.

I suppose it did look a bit odd when the four of us walked through the front door and three girls exclaimed, "Hey, Danno!" I had to explain that I'd known them for years through the radio show, and that reality was far more benign than perception.

However, had I walked in with a bunch of guys, I would have milked it like a Holstein.

Ironically, Stephanie's appearance that night fit the stereotypical Attitudes uniform. She was wearing tan work boots, corduroy pants, and—as an added bonus—a long-sleeve mock turtleneck with the word "HARDCORE" where a left breast pocket would live. Two minutes after she hit the dance floor, five horny women surrounded her.

Stephanie is from a small town in Illinois called Effingham, population twelve thousand. Effingham's lesbian club scene is not what you'd call vibrant. As far as Stephanie was concerned, these girls were just friendly, out for a night of dancing. I knew otherwise. I nearly took an elbow to the face (a deliberate jab, mind you) before they all turned to me, pissed at my presence. I was Peter Horton in *Children of the Corn*, and they were the female incarnations of Malachi, screaming "Outlander!" It was not pretty.

Stephanie spotted me across the floor, now bounced from the circle of estrogen. I'd like to think my sexy good looks drew her in; more likely, it was pity. Either way, she parted the ladies like Moses parting the Red Sea, walked right up to me, and kissed me. *En Francais*.

I threw my arms around her and we kissed passionately for a good two minutes. I don't think I breathed. Richard slipped a condom in my back pocket and smacked me on the bum. The music was pumping directly into my skull. I was dizzy, intoxicated by the raw, intense emotion of the moment. I'd never felt anything so real in my life.

And then she stopped.

"You have to walk away from me," she said.

I shook my head, not quite comprehending what I had just heard. "I…"

"You're leaving. Soon. I listen to the show every now and again."

I looked at her and sighed. She was right. I was leaving. Sometimes, reality sucks, even when you're making out on the dance floor in the middle of a lesbian nightclub. I nodded. I turned around and walked towards the bar, gutted by her honesty.

But then the strangest thing happened. A voice inside my head stated with audible authority, "If you walk away, you'll be making the biggest mistake of your life." Simple. Blunt. I turned around. She was still staring at me from the dance floor. I walked up to her and took her hand.

"I know I'm leaving, and I know you're here. I know I have no right to say this, but I really, really like you, and I'd like to make you happy for as long as I can. I'm not going to walk away unless you tell me to walk away."

"I can't."

And then, like clockwork, Richard sashayed up to us.

"Take me home. She doesn't want to share." And after a deep breath, "This is bullshit!"

He was not going to find a *ménage* at any point this evening. To him, the party was over. I looked at my watch. 2:05 a.m. I had to be at work in less than three hours.

As I pulled back into Schneithorst's parking lot, I said goodbye to Richard and his girlfriend and then turned to Stephanie. She was still not sober enough to drive safely, so I put on the full-court press.

"I'll take you back to my place. You can get an hour or two of sleep, I'll prepare for work, and I'll bring you back here on my way in. And I promise I won't try to take advantage of you."

She begrudgingly agreed. I found out later that this was truly an act of God. She'd never been to a guy's house on the first date. Ever.

We pulled up to the gate of my place, and I pushed the open button. She gave me a look that said, *You live here?* Thirty seconds later, I opened the garage door, revealing a Jaguar and a Mercedes. The next look: *What the hell do you do for a living besides radio?*

It wasn't that I'd hidden my situation from her. I just didn't think it would come up. Two weeks earlier, the lease was up on my apartment. Since I was going to leave in three months anyway, my parents offered to let me live at their house while I saved money on rent. It seemed perfectly logical.

What I had not expected, however, as I opened the door to the kitchen, was hearing the television. This meant only one thing: my mom was having stomach issues. She was probably drinking Pepto-Bismol and watching infomercials until she was tired enough to go back to bed.

She saw me walk in with Stephanie. I don't know which woman was more mortified. My mother apologized profusely.

"I'm so sorry!"

All I could do was laugh. It was the most ridiculous set of circumstances.

"Mom, I'd like you to meet Stephanie. Stephanie, this is my mom, Marie."

Without missing a beat, Stephanie gave my mother a firm handshake. "Nice to meet you."

After exchanging pleasantries, we said goodnight and headed upstairs.

"You better have a really good explanation for this."

I told her my story. Somehow, she believed it. We lay on the bed and talked for forty-five minutes. At one point during the conversation, she told me that she was Catholic, which prompted me to tell her that I loved a good fish fry. This prompted her to tell me that she always ate Captain D's once during Lent, "but it gives me diarrhea."

"Wow," was all I could think to say. She laughed.

"Probably shouldn't have told you that."

She was so fearless in knowing who she was. I was disarmed before I could put up a single defense. I was in trouble, and I knew it.

And I was okay with it. I gave her a peck on the cheek and told her to get some sleep. I'd be waking her soon enough. Then I sat down at my computer to write some sportscasts for the morning. Hitting the spacebar to pull up the screen, I leaned forward and touched my toes, rubbing my lower back with my hands.

The pain was getting worse.

# 3
# CHANGE OF PLANS

"What are you doing for Thanksgiving?"

"I'm going to my parents' house in Effingham."

It was our fourth official date, a lazy afternoon at the St. Louis Zoo. On a global scale, the St. Louis Zoo is one of the best. There are hundreds of species of animals from every continent, including bears, anacondas, giraffes, and the almost extinct Somali Wild Ass.

Exhibits include Big Cat Country with lions and tigers, the Penguin and Puffin Coast, and The River's Edge, where Stephanie and I found ourselves at that moment. The River's Edge boasts cheetahs, hyenas, a black rhino, hippos, and a full herd of Asian elephants. In fact, the St. Louis Zoo has one of the most successful elephant breeding programs on record. Which soon became obvious. We rounded a corner only to come face to face with the male's elephanthood. He was hung like a...well...elephant. We were utterly impressed.

"Effingham, huh?"

"Yes."

Stephanie spent every chance she could with her family, which is one of the things that drew me to her. She was exceptionally close to her parents, her brother, and her sister. She thought nothing of driving two hundred miles almost every weekend to visit for what amounted to little more than thirty-six hours.

"And what are you doing for Thanksgiving?" she asked.

Thanksgiving had never been one of the big holidays with my family. While it was always a nice night, the only thing I really remembered every year was watching the Macy's Thanksgiving Day Parade and eating dinner anywhere but our own house.

"Not sure. Richard said he's going to Hooters and asked if I wanted to go."

"Why don't you come home with me?"

We'd been together less than a month, and she just asked me not only to meet her parents, but to spend one of the big three holidays with them. *Holy shit*

"Where would I stay?"

"There's a guest room. Or if my Aunt Jean is there, you can sleep on the couch."

I was slightly terrified, but there was no way I was going to turn her invitation down. I really wanted to meet her parents and her siblings. I eagerly accepted. When I told my parents what I would be doing for Thanksgiving, they couldn't have been happier.

"Just don't miss Christmas."

I was a bundle of nerves during the drive to Effingham, which was ninety minutes from driveway to driveway. I would meet her parents, her brother, her sister, and her friends. Her parents would be "on their best behavior." Her friends "would love me." Her sister "is so much like her." Her brother?

"He may be a bit of a smart-ass. And a grump. And he'll be eyeing you up and down."

"Your brother a big guy?" I asked.

"No. But my dad is six-five."

"Lovely."

The next thing I knew, Stephanie and I were sitting on the floor of her parents' house, near the washer and dryer closet. Michele, her lovely mom, asked me about all sorts of things: where I came from, my parents, and my Irish heritage.

"I'm just an old Irish washer-woman, and it's great to have you here."

I loved her immediately.

That evening, Stephanie told me we would be seeing a legend of a local band called The Accousticats. They were playing the pre-Thanksgiving show at Sneaky Pete's, "which is all the way across town."

This always makes me giggle. In St. Louis, "all the way across town" means fighting traffic and road rage for thirty minutes as you try to get from point A to point B.

Sneaky Pete's was six minutes away on roads with speed limits topping off at 35 miles-per-hour.

"You could walk this," I remarked.

"You must be joking."

Before the concert, we grabbed some chicken wings at a bar called The Grey Dog. To this day, they are some of the best wings I've ever had. I don't know if it really was the sauce or simply Stephanie's presence.

While I was choking down my sixteenth wing, Stephanie's sister Courtney arrived. It took five wet-naps and an act of God to get clean enough to shake her hand, but I instantly fell in love with her, just as I had fallen in love with her mom. The three of us were soon engrossed in conversation that didn't let up for thirty minutes.

In the middle of our chat, Courtney lit up a cigarette. While still looking her in the eye, I walked sideways to the bar and grabbed an ashtray to bring back to the table. Stephanie later told me that this simple act of kindness was one of the things that endeared me to her—partially because I saw a need and filled it but mostly because of how I treated her sister.

*I know I'm going to L.A.*, I thought, *but it's going to suck hard to leave all of this.*

One hour and four beers later, Stephanie and Courtney were doing "the Train" on Sneaky Pete's dance floor. True to billing, The Accousticats were fantastic. One guitarist in particular, Larry, was exceptional. Larry would go on to play some pretty remarkable gigs, including *The Late Show with David Letterman* as part of The Fred Eaglesmith Traveling Steam Show.

This night was just getting better and better. Then Courtney spoke up.

"We forgot to gobble!"

"Gobble?"

## 3: CHANGE OF PLANS

I soon learned that "gobble" meant to gobble like a turkey before slamming a shot of Wild Turkey. I'm sure this beverage is palatable to a wide variety of tender, loving, caring people. However, I can only describe it as having Satan reach his fiery claw into my mouth, down my esophagus, and into my upper small intestine. While performing jazz hands.

Needless to say that when I woke up the next morning, I had absolutely no idea where I was, which sort of set the tone for Thanksgiving. The whole day was a whirlwind. At least twenty people crowded the house, which was filled with smells of turkey and stuffing and bread and vegetables. The aroma was intoxicating. Either that, or I was still intoxicated.

I finally met her dad, Dan, who had been at work when we left for the previous evening's festivities. Dan was huge, but he was also teddy-bearish, which meant I felt relatively safe.

The two people who stood out the most to me that day were Dan's parents. The minute Dan's dad discovered I worked in radio, the interrogation began.

"Why isn't there anything on 95.3?"

"How do you mean, sir?" I asked.

"There's a station on 95.5, but there is only static noise on 95.3. Why is that?"

"I'm guessing because there is no station residing at 95.3. You can only fit so many stations in one market," I said.

"But what causes the static?" he pressed.

"It's just electronic noise. There is no signal."

"But all I will need is an antenna to get rid of it?" he reasoned.

"An antenna will do nothing for you."

Stephanie mouthed the words "I'm sorry" while I stayed in his crosshairs.

"Well, what will an antenna do for me?" he asked.

"If you're getting your stations clearly, you don't need a new antenna."

"But if I had an antenna, could I pick up programming on 95.3?" he asked.

At this point, his wife couldn't take any more.

"I'd like to talk to the Irish boy if you'd just shut up!"

"I'm just asking him a question about radio!"

"Shut your jaw-jacking!"

At that moment, Steph's brother, Pat, walked up beside me, looked me in the eye, and said, "Welcome to the family, sir."

Just one week later, his words would become more profound than he knew.

—

"I'm sorry, but we require a jacket for the dining room," said the *maître d'* of Al's, one of the nicest St. Louis restaurants that no one has heard of. Located just outside a section of town called Laclede's Landing, which is known for loud college bars and even louder car sound-systems cruising its cobblestone streets, Al's boasts ridiculously good steaks.

And, apparently, a jacket requirement.

"I apologize. I had no idea," I stammered.

The night had not gotten off to the best of starts. I was twenty minutes late picking up Stephanie because I lost track of time in the shower.

And no, not because of what guys normally do to lose track of time in the shower.

My back had been at me for a few days. It was a nuisance, but sadly not uncommon. This was a big night, and I didn't want my malady to be a topic of conversation, so I did what I could to alleviate the pain. The quickest relief usually came from alternating between freezing cold and scalding hot water in the shower every two minutes or so. Apparently, I alternated a bit more than I had originally planned.

I also discovered that Stephanie and her family are sticklers for punctuality. This was an entirely foreign concept, as "sorry I'm late" were some of the first words I learned as a child. Whenever my parents invited me out to dinner, I'd be lucky to roll in by the appetizer. I had never even been to a baseball game before the fourth inning.

Yet there I was, tardy and jacketless. I was quickly in the hole 0 and 2.

"Not to worry, sir. It happens all the time. Please, come with me."

He led me to a room where several jackets hung, left unintentionally by inebriated patrons. I found a nice black one that I could have shared with a family of four. The guy who left it probably went home only to have his heart explode, God bless him. But it was either this or a knit one the color of vomit.

I returned to the table and took my seat. Dan looked at me and giggled.

"That would be big on me."

Again, disarmed by her parents. I loved these people. I loved her. It was real and unabashed. And it was frightening. Everything was changing, and I couldn't stop the train.

At one point, Stephanie and her mom stood up to use the restroom. Dan and I both stood up to wish them good luck. As we sat back down, he put his hand on my arm.

"Thank you for the way you treat my daughter."

I tried to think of something amazing or profound in response, but I was completely caught off guard. "You are welcome," I mustered.

"And please take care of her."

"I will, Dan."

Al's let me keep the jacket. I have no idea why. Stephanie and I drove back to her apartment. We were both silent, which was unlike us. Usually, the two of us never shut up. But my mind was racing faster than my heart. Was I really about to do what I was about to do?

"Do you mind if I take you somewhere? It's got a really good view."

In retrospect, I realize it probably sounded like code for "Do you mind if I kidnap and dismember you? No one will ever hear the scream."

Thankfully, she didn't take it that way. She accepted my invitation, and I drove to the top of a parking lot overlooking Clayton, a small city in St. Louis County that boasts a few skyscrapers of its own. The view is pretty impressive, especially with the twinkling lights of the burgeoning Christmas season percolating down the streets.

I pulled into the parking lot and drove to the top. We got out to look at the lights. The temperature was dropping, so I put my new sport-tent (courtesy of Al's) around her.

"Aren't you cold?" she asked.

Actually, I was sweating. "No, I'm all good."

We were quiet for a while.

"It was a wonderful night," she finally ventured. "My parents really like you. They're going to miss you."

"Stephanie, I love you, and I can't leave you." There, I said it.

"What?"

"I can't leave you. I love you. I'm not going to Los Angeles. I can't. I'd be nothing without you."

"Dan, this is your dream. I can't ask you to do that."

"You didn't. I've been thinking about this since the night we kissed. You're it. You are what makes me happy. L.A. can wait."

Her expression was filled with competing emotions. *Did that just happen? Did he tell me he loves me? What did he just give up for me? Do I tell him I love him? Do I love him? Wait, of course I love him. Don't be silly. Is this what I want? What do I do? What do we do? What comes next? He looks so sexy in this light and I'm going to attack him.* (Okay, maybe not that last one.)

"Are you sure about this?" she asked.

"I've never been so sure about anything in my life," I said. "I love you."

"I love you." There, she said it. There was no going back.

# 4

## DOESN'T EVER LEAVE THE AIRPORT

I was born in Dublin, Ireland, on September 1st, 1972. Not that I gave it a whole lot of thought as a child, but I figured that I would spend my entire life in my homeland. However, life does have a funny way of shaking you out of complacency. Imagine our surprise when my dad came home one day and said, "We're moving to America."

"What do you mean *we*, Raymond?" asked my mother.

My dad was being given the opportunity to help Jefferson Smurfitt Corporation, the company he worked for, expand their foothold in the United States. He was thrilled. Marie was pissed.

It would mean leaving her mother and sister, all of our extended family, and the only life she ever knew. The fact that the decision was made without consulting her was that little added "something" that made it even less palatable. How my father talked her into going is the stuff of legend.

When the four of us arrived in the United States in 1977, my mother and father made a pact: she would raise my brother Gavin and me, and he would try to earn as much money as possible so that their children would not have to struggle growing up like they did. It was not the easiest life, but they succeeded.

While my parents loved each other, the arrangement was hard on both of them. My mother not only had the unenviable task of raising two boys alone (most of the time), but she also resented my father for eating great food and drinking great wine and being a captain of industry, just for "pushing a fucking pen!"

My father resented the fact that my mother resented him and didn't care to understand how hard he worked. "I do not push a pen!"

What my mother had not realized was that after almost two decades of this understanding, she had grown accustomed to her lifestyle. She liked her time to herself and was fiercely protective of it. I learned this on the night my father retired. My dad worked in two places for the same company: the purely corporate side in the Smurfitt Tower in Clayton, Missouri, and the Smurfitt I.T. department in Alton, a river town across the Mississippi in Illinois, and home to the tallest man who ever lived, Robert Wadlow, the Alton Giant.

Both sets of employees loved my dad. He treated the most blue-collar worker and the most white-collar worker with the same level of respect. Smart businessman, my father.

## 4: DOESN'T EVER LEAVE THE AIRPORT

On the night of his going-away dinner in Alton, I sat with my mom as my dad gave a speech. It was eloquent and heartfelt, and it ended with, "And now that I'm retired, I'm going to be spending a lot more time at home with Marie."

I may have been the only one in the crowd who heard it. It was faint, reflexive. It was only because we sat beside each other that I heard my mother mutter a distinct, "Oh, shit."

After years of lamenting to me that he should just quit that damn job, it finally happened. As the reality set in that she was stuck with him, she learned that she couldn't get the genie back in the bottle, no matter what the storybooks say.

Marie was all out of wishes.

Two weeks later, she bought him a set of golf clubs and said, "Get out of my house."

So my father took up golf, and he used his new skills to beat the tar out of my brother and me every Christmas and New Year in Bermuda.

I admit that a trip to Bermuda is an odd Christmas tradition, but it worked for us. When we first moved to the United States, it was just the four of us. The rest of our family was across the Atlantic Ocean. The one time that we did go back to Ireland for Christmas, we said goodbye to my dad's dad (who was dying of cancer), and we spent a few hours at the hospital with my mom's mom (who got hit by a car).

After one last frigid Christmas alone in St. Louis, my parents had had enough.

"Screw this, we're going to the beach," said my father.

Remember, we're Irish. We're fair skinned, and we burn easily. We wanted to go to a beach, but we also didn't want to go anywhere where the sun would be too intense. Bermuda fit the bill.

Plus, we had been there once before, and we had liked it. Now that my parents could afford to stay where they wanted, it became our Christmas home.

Ray and Marie offered to pay for Stephanie to join us that Christmas of 2001, but she was reticent.

"I think it's too soon. And my parents are pretty conservative, so they might have an issue with you and I staying in a hotel together."

As much as I looked forward to the thought of hanging out with Steph in a bikini, I understood her argument. When I told my folks this, they were blown out of the water. And then they did something that blew me out of the water: they told me that since Steph declined, I could ask a friend to go. My brother would be there with his wife, which meant I would be on my own for the ten-day trip.

I called my friend Richard.

"Dude, how'd you like to go to Bermuda with us?"

"Whose dick would I have to suck to get to do that?" Richard is never at a loss for words.

Three days after Christmas, I met him at Wade International Airport in St. George's, Bermuda. We rode the forty-five minutes back to our hotel on my rented scooter. My back was killing me, but thankfully the adrenaline kept my agony at bay.

I had my best friend with me for six days in my favorite place on earth. We would play golf and tennis. We would scuba dive and swim with dolphins. We would explore the island on scooters and eat like kings and do shots. It was like a honeymoon, without the cuddling. We were going to have a fantastic vacation, pain be damned.

On day one, I played golf with my dad while Richard slept in. Then we had breakfast. Then we played tennis. Then we went exploring on the scooters. Then we found a pharmacy because Bermuda pharmacies sell Tylenol with Codeine over the counter. Then we had dinner. Then we played Bingo. Then I passed out.

On day two, I played golf with my dad while Richard slept in. Then we had breakfast. Then we went to the pool. Then we went exploring on the scooters. Then I spent two hours in a fetal position in a bathtub because I couldn't walk. Then we ate dinner. Then I swallowed the last four of the sixteen Advil Liquigels I would take that day. Then I passed out.

On day three, I played golf with my dad. Richard…no. Then we had breakfast. Then we explored on the bikes. Then we went scuba diving. Then we took showers and got ready for our New Year's Eve dinner. Then we sat down at the table at The Newport Room, the nicest restaurant I've ever seen. Then the appetizers came. Then I ate one shrimp…

And then I excused myself from the table. And I looked at my parents and at my brother Gavin and his wife Alison and at Richard. "I can't do this anymore," I said. "Goodnight."

And then I went up to the room. And then I popped the last four of the sixteen Advil I would take that day. And then I called Stephanie to wish her a Happy New Year and to tell her I loved her and to tell her that aside from her not being there, I was having the time of my life. And then I got naked, got into the tub, curled up into a ball, asked God to take away my pain by any means necessary, and passed out.

I don't know how boxers ended up on my body or how I moved from the tub to the bed.

On day four, we explored the island. On day five, we called a friend in St. Louis to get the number of a back surgeon. On day six, we swam with the dolphins at Dolphin Quest before heading to the airport. It was a great trip, and I was finally going to see Stephanie in a few hours. All was right with the world. Pain be damned.

—

"Ladies and gentlemen, please remain in your seats. The taxiway is a mess, and we're not going anywhere anytime soon. Please sit back and relax."

The pilot's voice clicked off as we came to a stop near the runway at Hartsfield Jackson International Airport in Atlanta. The city was caught in a freak snowstorm. By the time it ended, the city was buried beneath a solid four inches of snow. In New England, that's a dusting. In the South, it's a blizzard, y'all.

We had already been in the air for over two hours. Once the plane landed, we didn't move a single inch for another two hours. I called my parents in Bermuda on my rapidly dying cell phone to let them know the situation and to alert them that, in six minutes, we were going to miss our connecting flight. I also called Stephanie to tell her not to wait up. There wasn't a sliver of a chance in hell that I would get home by midnight.

Nearly three hours after we landed, our plane made it to the jet bridge. The pain in my back was so severe I could barely stand up out of my seat. I don't know how I maneuvered my way down the aisle to disembark.

The first thing I needed was Advil. I had exhausted my supply mid-flight. I could take four more before the end of the day, and I was going to suck down every last one of them as fast as I could. And then I would go to bed—wherever that meant. We were stuck in Atlanta. In a snowstorm.

# 4: DOESN'T EVER LEAVE THE AIRPORT

My brother had other ideas.

"I don't want to stay in this airport one minute longer than I have to. I want to go home."

We all did. So did everyone else on our flight. Fortunately, my brother Gavin is a little guy, and he was able to weave his way through the pugilistic crowd at the ticket counter and cut to the front of the line.

"Dan! Get over here!"

Gavin, our personal Houdini, turned a wait that should have taken hours into a mere four minutes. And as his final trick, he sweet-talked the gate agent into getting the four of us on the last flight to St. Louis. It was scheduled for 8:45 p.m. Maybe I would get home before midnight!

With a couple of hours to kill, we grabbed a bite to eat. (After I took some Advil, that is.) My brother's wife, Alison, was not feeling well. She was two months pregnant, and we chalked up her queasiness to the pregnancy. At any rate, the stress of the afternoon would have made anyone feel lousy. But there was a cure: T.G.I. Friday's potato skins. I devoured two full portions. Then I cursed myself for making the pain worse. Potato skins cure a lot of things. Like depression. And hunger. They're not so effective for searing back pain.

By 9:00 p.m., the snow still hadn't stopped. It appeared we weren't going anywhere, despite Houdini's antics. Resigned would-be passengers began booking every last hotel room within a ten-mile radius. But at 9:20, our saving grace arrived by way of a message from the gate attendant over the loudspeaker: "Ladies and gentlemen, we will now begin our boarding process for our non-stop flight to St. Louis."

"Thank you, God," my brother mumbled.

We were going home.

Because we were the last people to secure seats on the flight, we weren't able to sit together. Some kind-hearted passengers moved around so Gavin and Alison could sit together. Richard and I simply said, "See you in St. Louis."

The cabin door was closed, and the flight attendant's voice came across the speaker system to inform us that we would be backing away from the gate at approximately 9:45 p.m. and would hit the de-icing pad shortly thereafter.

This would not be the first lie told to us that night.

By 11:00 p.m., we hadn't budged. Some passengers had already fallen asleep. I hadn't. I've never been able to sleep on a plane, and the pain was like an added jolt of caffeine. The few passengers who remained awake started grumbling. At 11:30, the pilot's voice came over the loudspeaker.

"Folks, one of the de-icing machines is broken, so they're having to make do with only one. There are about twelve planes ahead of us. Once we make our way to the pad, it should only take about twenty minutes to de-ice before we're cleared for takeoff. I'm guessing it's going to be about two hours."

Lie #2. There was an audible groan from the passengers.

At 1:30 a.m., our plane backed up from the gate. *Finally!* I thought. The plane moved fifty feet. And then stopped. It did not move for another hour. No one said anything to us. There was no food or water. The imprisoned passengers grew increasingly agitated.

At 2:40 a.m., our plane moved again, made a turn, and headed towards the de-icing pad. Or so we thought. It taxied another two hundred feet. And stopped moving. This time, we didn't move again until 4:00. Cell phones were long dead. The crewmembers were no longer speaking. And I don't have a single word that can possibly describe my pain at that moment.

Lie #3. By omission.

At 4:20 a.m., we made it to the de-icing pad, where nothing happened for thirty-five minutes.

At 4:55 a.m., the workers started the de-icing process. If you've never seen it, it's a bit unnerving. Men with water cannons blast every inch of the plane with a chemical to make sure that ice doesn't form on the wings during flight, which could drop your plane out of the sky like a boulder, Wyle. E. Coyote style. The whole process takes about thirty minutes.

In the middle of getting hosed, the pilot addressed his prisoners once more. He sounded cheerful. Bastard.

"Folks, this is your captain speaking. Hopefully, after the de-icing, we'll get out of here and on up to St. Louis."

Lie #4.

At 5:25 a.m., after we were properly de-iced, the plane started moving out onto the taxiway. We were finally going home.

Ha.

We cleared the de-icing pad, and the plane stopped. Forty minutes passed. We didn't move. We had been on the road to nowhere for over eight hours. The crew was nowhere to be seen. There was still no food or water. All cell phones were dead. No one talked.

At 5:58 a.m., the plane started to move. And then…

"Ladies and gentlemen, this is your captain speaking. Due to FAA regulations, crews may only work certain time limits. We are, unfortunately, going to have to turn back to the gate and let you off."

The plane was silent. No one said anything. Not…one…thing. We made it to the gate in six minutes. I stood for the first time in almost nine hours and nearly fell into the aisle. I grabbed my bag. Almost every single passenger gave the crew an earful on the way out.

"Bastards."

"You did this just so you wouldn't have to buy us hotel rooms."

"I'm going to sue you."

"How dare you!"

"I can't believe you did this to us."

"What kind of people do this to other people?"

"Thanks for the rape."

I didn't say anything. I was in too much pain. I just looked at them and shook my head. I wanted to waggle my finger at them, but that might have been overkill.

We scanned the tarmac from inside the terminal. Hartsfield is already one of the busiest airports in the world. Getting home within the next twenty-four hours was not a guarantee. I looked at my three traveling buddies.

"Screw this," I said. "I know the way home from here. Let's rent a car and drive it."

After trying unsuccessfully to retrieve our bags back from the airline, we abandoned our luggage, rented a minivan, found a local Sprint store to purchase phone chargers, and drove nine hours home. Our bags arrived the next day.

# 5

# THE RED HERRINGS

In the 1991 movie *JFK*, in one of my favorite scenes in cinematic history, Donald Sutherland's X tells Kevin Costner's Jim Garrison, "That's the real question isn't it. Why? The how and the who is just scenery for the public. Oswald. Ruby. Cuba. The Mafia. Keeps 'em guessing like some kind of parlor game, prevents 'em from asking the most important question: why?"

I spent hours upon hours trying to figure out "the why" of so much agony. There were many culprits.

From my early days in utero, I have not had the best of lower backs. In my lowest lumbar, the one above my tailbone, there is scar tissue where bone should reside. I found this out when I started playing a lot of tennis in high school. One wrong back hand, and I'd be out of commission. This would last a few days, and then my vertebrae would invariably work their way back into place. As I got older, however, these episodes became more acute, especially when I added golf to the menu. My mom told me to seek relief from her chiropractor, Dr. Scott Bakunas.

Dr. Bakunas beat the living hell out of my lower back, wrenching it back into place. It was not the most comfortable experience, but it seemed to do the trick. He was exceptionally good at his craft, so much so that I thought I'd never have any back issues again.

Then one day while disrobing for a shower, I took off a pair of white boxers. As they fell to the floor, I noticed a small stain about an inch below the waistband. It looked out of place that high up, and it didn't look like anything that is usually produced by that part of the body. This looked more like the remnants in a chewing tobacco dip cup.

But I'm a boy, and I chalked it up to a possible rogue shart.

Over the next three days, I saw the exact same stain in the exact same spot on my boxers. It was unnerving. I groped my lower back to see if I could feel anything odd. At first, nothing seemed out of the ordinary. Then, I found a small indentation at the very top of my butt crack. I probed it with my finger and looked at my hand.

Tobacco juice. *What the hell!*

I immediately called my doctor and told him what was going on.

"Dan, it sounds like a Pilonidal cyst," he said.

"A what?"

"An ingrown hair."

## 5: THE RED HERRINGS

Once upon a time, several years earlier, a very small hair at my lower back popped out. Perhaps it was a cold day, perhaps he was shy, but for some reason, he decided to go back the way he came. He made a new hole with his microscopically spiky head and crawled back in. He grew strong and long. Probably played football in high school. And then the jerk wrapped himself around my tailbone and lowest vertebra. Over and over and over again. Who does that? *What* does that?

Basically, I was sporting an epic comb-over directly beneath my butt skin.

It was an uneventful surgery, save for the moment I woke up in the middle of it. I was lying on my belly when I opened my eyes. I turned my head and looked up at the surgeon, who had now completely stopped what he was doing. We locked gazes.

"Wwwwwwhat are you doing, doc?" I asked.

"Uh…I'm sewing you up, Dan," he replied.

"Ahhhhh…okay." And then I went back to sleep. Apparently, it's true what they say: redheads need more anesthesia than non-gingers.

The cyst had grown so large that the surgeon had to make a "V" at the top of my butt crack to dig it out. When he sewed me up, the incision made a very small "cheek" between my two larger cheeks. Yes, I now had a third butt cheek, but my I was fixed.

Then in my early twenties, my back started to treat me fifty ways to wrong. I called up my Mom's long-lost chiropractor and asked him to break it into submission. He agreed. I saw him two days later.

He started my treatment with some x-rays, which proved yet another reason why my back gave me fits. The holes in the sides of my vertebrae, the tunnels that allow my tubes and wires to meander through that part of my body, were significantly smaller than they should have been, which meant my nerves were getting crimped. The weaker my back was, the worse the crimping became. Dr. Bakunas instructed me to strengthen my core. He gave me a green rubber ball the size of Delaware and prescribed five minutes of bouncing per day.

The big green ball seemed to do the trick. Sure, I felt goofy bouncing on this thing like a six-year-old on a red bouncy elephantitic testicle with the rubber handle, but my back decompressed, improving my situation dramatically. I was finally free from pain.

And then, October 21, 1996, happened.

I was two and a half years into my radio career with *Steve and DC*. I had finally built up my reputation as a sportscaster enough to have a bar in St. Charles, Missouri, offer me a Monday Night Football remote.

Remotes are the lifeblood of disc jockeys. You show up at a public event, hang out, and get paid better than billable hours at a law firm. At the height of their popularity, Steve and DC actually made more from remotes than they did from their salaries, which were impressive in their own right.

My job was to hang out at the bar from 8:00 until 11:00 p.m. and call the station twice an hour to ballyhoo the location, food and drink specials, and prizes we were giving away. The rest of the time, I was welcome to eat, drink, and chat with the listeners. In turn, they would pay me more money in three hours than I made in an entire week.

The first two weeks of the remotes were pristine. The bar manager was happy, the place was packed, I was connecting with some of our biggest fans, and I was making fat bank. The potato

# 5: THE RED HERRINGS 49

skins were pretty fabulous, as well (though not as good as T.G.I. Fridays). The only perk I denied myself was liquor. I learned early in my radio career that even a single beer makes waking up at 3:30 a.m. way harder than it needs to be. Coca Cola became my beverage of choice. At first, the listeners were slightly upset with this: "What do you mean you won't do the Three Wise Men shot I just bought for you?" Then I'd explain my situation, and they'd buy me a Coke instead. I drank a lot of caffeine in those first two weeks.

For week three of the Monday Night Football remote, I went to the mall to buy a new blue sweater—St. Louis Rams blue—at Mark Shale. Sure, Mr. Shale was a little expensive, but I could afford it at this point. I took a nap, ate dinner, attended a quick meeting about an upcoming Halloween broadcast, and headed to the bar.

The night was uneventful. The call-ins went well, the people were nice, I limited myself to five Cokes, and the potato skins were as scrumptious as ever. I waved goodbye to the crowd and made my way to my Jeep Wrangler, Daisy.

Black as night with fat wheels, a monster sound system, and a brush guard that looked like Darth Vader's dentures, Daisy was the love of my life. I had driven her for five years, but I still felt a rush every time I looked at her. She was my baby.

Her only drawback was her little four-banger engine. She was really quick up to thirty miles-per-hour, but after that, she could maybe make it to sixty if you were going downhill in a tail wind while stroking the shifter and talking dirty to her. Maybe.

I had been on the road for approximately eight minutes. It was a cloudy night, but not all that cold for late October. The window on my soft top was zipped down. The sound system was pumping.

Interstate 70 was a little busy for 11:00 p.m., and traffic was not faster than fifty miles-per-hour. I was tired and needed to get to bed. I saw an opening in the fast lane, next to a tractor-trailer. I pulled into the lane and threw Daisy into fourth gear. My foot was buried to the floor. Slowly, she began creeping past the rig.

I didn't like being in the fast lane with her. Her engine just couldn't handle it. I looked across at the truck. My back tires were parallel with its grill. *Almost there.*

I turned my head back towards the road. That's when I heard a piercing screech behind me. As my eyes shot up to my rearview mirror, I saw two headlights blow up like fireworks. The approaching car had already slammed on its breaks and the wheels were locked, but it was going too fast to slow down.

"Oh, shit."

I clung to the dashboard with my right hand and the steering wheel with the left. Half a second later, *impact*. The smack of metal on metal was shockingly loud. Daisy's back end fishtailed. I grabbed the wheel with both hands to try to steer out of it, but to no avail.

Daisy and I were on the shoulder, sliding helplessly towards the concrete barrier that separated the eastbound and westbound lanes of Interstate 70. The Missouri Department of Transportation—MO DOT—had installed what they called "flip walls" along this stretch of the highway. The flip walls prevented runaway drivers from crossing into oncoming lanes and potentially crashing head-first into a car coming the opposite way.

I can't explain what occurred next. The laws of physics and geometry prove inadequate.

As Daisy spun around and hit the wall, she started flipping. I clenched the steering wheel for dear life, only to feel my hands let

## 5 : THE RED HERRINGS

go—inexplicably—and my arms raise up and out of the unzipped windows. It was as though I was pulled out of the Jeep, mid-flip, by my wrists.

I flew backwards at sixty miles-per-hour, facing up, four feet off the ground. I watched Daisy flip wildly as I soared away from her. The windshield exploded. The ground tore away the convertible soft top. CD's streaked through the sky like tiny silver Frisbees, as if they were launched out of a skeet flinger.

Oh look, *The Innocents* by Erasure.

*Pull!*

And in the midst of the chaos, a composed voice popped into my head: "Dan, keep your head up." I flew backwards, my back to the street; keeping my head up meant planting my chin to my chest, which is exactly what I did.

Less than a half-second later, I hit the ground. At sixty miles-per-hour.

My shoulders grazed the pavement first. I smacked the asphalt two more times, like a rock across a lake. I did not roll or tumble. My body simply skipped.

After the third collision with the ground, my inertia ceased. I looked up at the sky. The tractor-trailer had stopped to my left. The flip wall was on my right. I lay dead-center on a six-foot-wide shoulder. If my trajectory had been two inches to the right, I would have hit the wall headfirst. Two inches to my left would have sent my body into the path of the tractor-trailer. Two inches lower and the back of my head would have been ripped off my body.

*What the hell just happened?*

I stood up. My hip was sore, as was my right shoulder blade. I had a small bump on the back of my head.

And my new sweater was slightly torn. *Son of a...*

These realizations came slowly as I walked towards Daisy, who was now upside-down. The roll cage had collapsed in the front; if I had stayed in the car, my head and torso would have been crushed. One of her back wheels was still spinning. *Where Do You Go* by No Mercy was still pumping through the subs. *Cashmere* by Led Zeppelin would have been a cooler choice, but you can't always get what you want (which would have been another good option).

The man who hit me was already out of his car, screaming.

"Oh, my God! Holy shit! Are you alright? Holy shit! Oh, my God! Oh, my God!"

"Could you please shut up?" I was in no mood to hear a single word he had to say.

"Yes! Oh, my God! I'm so sorry! Oh, my God!"

Tim, my co-worker who had been at the bar with me and who may have been three sheets to the wind, witnessed the whole crash from his own vehicle. It must have been horrific. He jumped out of his car, walked up to me, stared into my eyes, and then walked over to Daisy. Crouching down on his hands and knees, he peered through the window.

He was looking for my body. He had, after all, just seen my ghost.

"Tim, can I use your phone?"

Still ashen and unconvinced that I was not an apparition, Tim handed me his phone. I called 9-1-1 and told them where I was. Apparently, I was the twenty-third person to call within the span of two minutes. The entire highway had stopped. The debris field enveloped five lanes of traffic. People were out of their cars. They didn't want to look at the dead body they thought they'd see, but they couldn't look away.

"Can I make another call?" I asked.

"Yeah, sure."

Tim put his hand on my shoulder. Yes, I was real.

"Hello?"

"Mom, it's me. I'm okay, but I've been in an accident and I'm headed to St. John's." I didn't want my parents to find out about this on the air.

"Are you hurt?" My mother was trying not to panic.

"I'm a little sore, but otherwise, I'm in great shape," I lied.

The ambulance arrived to take me away for testing and observation. They put me on a backboard on the side of the road while I protested.

"Is all of this necessary?"

The medic looked at the mangled wreck and then back at me. "Are you kidding me, kid?"

They strapped me to the backboard, placed the backboard on a gurney, and pushed the gurney into the ambulance.

"Please take me to St. John's. I told my mom I was going to St. John's."

St. John's Mercy Hospital was not just around the corner. The paramedics offered to take me to a closer hospital, but I was adamant. It was the first time I had ever been so vocal about my own healthcare. I was glad I stood my ground.

They asked me which body parts hurt. My hip was sore. I had a headache. The back of my right shoulder stung quite a bit. As soon as I said the bit about my shoulder, the paramedic whipped out a pair of scissors. He was going to cut my new St. Louis Rams blue sweater.

"Dude, I just bought this today. I can take it off."

Again, he shook his head at me.

Snip. Snip. Snip. Snip.

"Ohhh," said the paramedic.

"What, ohhhhh?" I asked.

He looked at his partner. "Tweezers."

The paramedic then picked a small chunk of Interstate 70 out of my shoulder. The pain was phenomenal, and the Betadine he mopped me with made it look like my shoulder and neck were covered in dried blood.

*Must not let my mother see me like this,* I thought.

Two hours later, as I lay on the backboard at the hospital, an officer arrived and said it was a miracle I survived. The accident reconstruction showed that the car that hit me had slowed down to just over one hundred miles-per-hour at the point of impact.

"Was he drunk?" I asked.

"No. He'd just gotten off work at the casino. New car, too. Still had temp stickers on the windows. Probably wanted to see how fast it would go."

"I can tell you how fast it stopped."

The officer laughed and headed to the door. He turned around and smiled. "You're here for a reason, kid."

I was a twenty-four-year-old male who had just lived through a smash-up that should have killed me ten different ways.

I knew my reason for being there.

*I was invincible.*

---

March 2, 2002. Advil had stopped working weeks before. Baths did nothing. The epidural steroid injection I received in February wore off less than two days after it was administered. It hurt to stand. It hurt to sit. It hurt to drive. It hurt to sleep. It hurt to eat. Without even trying, I dropped thirty pounds.

I curled up in a ball and rocked on my left side. I was terrified. I had no idea what was wrong with me, and I prayed with everything I had.

"God, I can't see my life this way for another ten years. I'm twenty-nine. I should not feel like this. Please take the pain away from me in any way you can, even if it means I have to die. I can't do this anymore."

I stood up and almost fell over. I grabbed my cell phone and called my chiropractor.

"Hello?"

"Scott, it's Dan." I was almost in tears.

"Danny, what's wrong?"

"I can't take this anymore, man. I don't know what to do."

"I hear ya, pal. Do you wanna come in?"

"I don't think I can drive."

"Okay. Well, we've gotta loosen up that lower back. Are you near a bed?"

"Uh huh."

"Okay, I want you to sit on the bed and then lie down while keeping your feet on the floor."

While much easier said than done, I was able to do as he asked.

"Now what?"

"Now I want you to put down the phone, and I want you to slowly bring your right knee up to your chest and hold it for thirty seconds. Then I want you to slowly bring it down. Then do the same for the left side. Can you do that?"

"I think so."

I put the phone down beside me on the bed and did as he had instructed. I slowly brought my right knee up to my chest and held it for half a minute. It did provide a little relief. I lowered my right leg and began to bring my left leg up.

And then, something moved in my abdomen. At first, the jabbing sensation was subtle, but the higher my knee came up, the more intense the dagger felt. I lowered my knee to the point where the pain subsided, and then I brought it up a few inches and then down a few inches. I could definitely feel something move.

"Scott, I'm going to call you back."

I didn't wait for his response.

# 6

## THE TIP OF MY ICEBERG

"That shouldn't be there."
I said the words out loud. My fingertips probed what seemed to be a lump the size of a golf ball about an inch below the left side of my rib cage. I was shocked. A lump? Seriously?

I knew my mother would lose her mind; I couldn't tell her. I knew my dad would tell my mom; I couldn't tell him either. My friends were…well…

I would have told Stephanie, but she was at work, and it wouldn't have been a good time. So I kept my Titleist-sized invader to myself for the next six hours.

Stephanie got off work early that day, and we headed to Effingham to see her parents. I didn't want to miss the visit, so I held my tongue during the entire drive. We chatted about her work, my work, the weather, and our plans for the night. I didn't say anything about what I had found.

Later that evening, Stephanie's parents left for church. She and I sat on the couch in their family room, kissing, telling each other how in love we were. And it was young love. We had been together a grand total of four months plus one day. Yet behind my happiness, I hid the most genuine worry I'd had in years. I had to tell her about the lump, and I did so in the only way I knew how: clumsily blurting it out.

"Steph, I was having some pain today and I called Scott and he gave me an exercise to try and I felt something move in my abdomen and I found a lump."

I felt like Ralphie asking Santa for a gun in *A Christmas Story*.

"Say that again?" she asked (read: gently demanded).

"I found a lump."

I took her hand, and I brought it right to the spot. She probed it intently, leaning her face down for a closer look.

"Dan, that shouldn't be there."

"I know."

"Have you seen a doctor yet?"

"I just found it a few hours ago."

"Dan, you have to see a doctor about this."

"I haven't had a doctor in years."

"Go to a Doc-in-the-Box."

Stephanie had borrowed this term from my mother, who did not have a regular doctor in a regular medical building. She preferred the staff at the local Urgent Care just up the street from their house.

"I'll go to my mom's guy on Monday."

"Do you promise?" Stephanie was adamant.

"Yes, I promise."

—

The doctor felt up and down the right side of my abdomen, digging his fingers into the nooks and crannies of my intestines.

"Does this hurt?"

"I can't say it's comfortable."

He kept staring at my abdomen, probing his hands towards the left side. He pushed down and dug his fingers in for about a second when he found the culprit.

"Hmmm. That shouldn't be there."

"I didn't think so," I replied.

"Give me a moment." He left the room.

*Maybe he's fetching a huge needle to lance what could be the biggest boil in human history! Maybe he's filling a bottle of Amoxicillin for the infection.* My mind sifted through the implausible options in a brief moment of levity. *It's all so ridiculous.*

The doctor came back into the room. No hacksaw. No pills. He simply handed me a piece of paper with two names and two numbers.

"Call one of them. I'm afraid this is beyond my scope."

Hello, fear. It's been a while.

—

"I'm sorry, but he's not accepting new patients for two weeks." The gatekeeper on the other end had her orders down pat.

"But ma'am," I pleaded, "I found a lump in my abdomen."

"I'm sorry sir, but the doctor is not accepting new patients for two weeks."

Had she heard a single word I said? God only knows what was going on in my body, and all she could do was parrot the company line. Angry, I hurled a four-letter expletive and hung up the phone.

I felt my abdomen again to make sure that I was not making this up. *Still there. Shit.*

I picked up the piece of paper again. It was time to dial doctor number two, Dr. Richard Pennell at St. John's.

"Dr. Pennell's office."

"Hi, I got your number from another doctor and I need to make an appointment."

"I'm sorry, but the doctor is not seeing any new patients for three weeks."

"Oh my God," I mumbled, crippled with fear.

But this time, the gatekeeper cracked. Barely.

"What's your medical issue?" Her voice had softened.

"I...I...found a lump in my abdomen."

"Hold."

For two minutes, I sat in complete silence. I could hear my own heartbeat in my eardrums. Every hair on my body stood up. My palms started to sweat. My breathing became shallow. And then, out of nowhere, somebody hit play on the *Jeopardy!* theme song in my head. I started whistling, and I couldn't stop.

Just when I hummed the concluding *boam! boam!*, the phone came to life.

"Can you be here tomorrow at nine?"

## 6: THE TIP OF MY ICEBERG

"Absolutely."

—

Dr. Richard Pennell was a man in his late forties and a bit old school with a white coat and a red tie. I liked him immediately. Except for his hands, which were exceptionally cold as they pushed and prodded and plucked and pointed and pinched every millimeter of my golf ball.

"I'm guessing you know this shouldn't be there," he said.

"I've heard that."

"Give me a minute."

Usually, when a doctor asks you to give him a minute, he heads out the door, maybe has a snack or a bathroom break (or so I imagine). Not Dr. Pennell. He held nothing back. He picked up the phone in the exam room, pushed a button, listened for a few moments, and said, "Put me through to radiology."

It's always odd to hear only one side of a conversation. It's unnerving when that conversation occurs in a doctor's office. It's heart-pounding when the topic of discussion is you.

"Hi, it's Richard. I need a CT. [pause] Immediately. [pause] Not good enough. [pause] It's urgent. [pause] It's for me. [pause] Got it. Thank you."

Dr. Pennell hung up the phone and looked me in the eye, not blinking, not averting his gaze.

"Mr. Duffy, I'm not gonna lie. This is pretty serious. You've got an emergency CT scan tomorrow at eight. You'll come back in here at 9:00 a.m. on Thursday for the results."

—

"This is going to feel a little hot."

The radiology assistant performing my CT scan pushed a plunger of contrast dye into my blood stream. Contrast dye is used to find anomalies in the body, and it is responsible for a trifecta of fun.

The first stage involves a gallon of putrid yogurt. Technically, it's not a gallon, but the unpalatable cocktail comes in a handle jug filled to the brim, and it can top off two very large Styrofoam cups with a bit to spare. You have to drink every last drop within the space of twenty minutes before the scan. It's also not yogurt, per se, but it is by far the thickest white liquid I've ever had the displeasure of choking down.

The active ingredient is barium. If that sounds familiar, it may have to do with that one time when you were a kid and your parents gave you a barium enema so you could poop. Colon exfoliation is the third and final stage of this journey of suck.

But stage two is by far the worst. Stage two is when the contrast dye works its infernal magic. I'd heard the sensation described as every cell in your body blushing at the same time. It doesn't quite feel like that. Instead, imagine a sunburn beneath your skin spontaneously ignites, starting with your extremities. The flames migrate from your fingers and toes, up your legs, down your arms, and through your torso—and end at your anus.

Yes, I said it: your butthole bursts into flames.

"You have to stop moving," the nurse admonished me for the fifth time.

"You try keeping still while your ass is on fire!" I wanted to yell. But I held my tongue like the good Catholic boy my mother raised me to be. I bit my lip and focused on my body as it was shuttled slowly into the whirring machine. I hadn't had a CT scan since October 22, 2006. I couldn't help but think that the two tests were somehow related.

—

*Click.*

My mom stopped in the middle of her fifth Hail Mary of her second decade of the Rosary. My dad's eyes shifted from me to the door. I turned my head in the same direction. Someone had hung the clipboard outside the room. There would finally be an answer. I looked at my parents as I slid off the examination table.

"I have to know."

I opened the door and started reading the clipboard. I didn't understand most of it until I reached the middle paragraph.

"Huge…encapsulating organs…possible lymphoma," I read.

"Possible what?" asked my father.

"Lymphoma. That's cancer, isn't it?" I'd heard of lymphoma, but I wasn't sure exactly what it meant.

The color drained from my mother's face. My father took her hand and rested his head against hers. I read the words over and over in disbelief.

Possible lymphoma.

Lymphoma.

Lymphoma.

I heard footsteps approaching down the hallway. I didn't want to get caught with my hand in the possibly cancerous cookie jar. Shuffling back to the examination table, I hopped up as Dr. Pennell walked through the door. He shook my hand and then the hands of my parents.

"Good morning," he said. He didn't smile.

"It's bad, isn't it?" I asked.

"It's big, that's for sure. Have you been having symptoms?"

"A lot of back pain."

"That doesn't surprise me. This thing is the size of a football."

"Holy shit, are you serious?" At this point, pleasantries went out the window.

"Unfortunately. It's wrapped around your left kidney, just below your lung. It's pushing your spine sideways trying to find more room."

"More room for what?" I asked.

"To grow. My guess is it's been growing for the better part of a year."

Steve's pool party. The drop to my knees. The recurring pain. Things started to make sense (not including my inexplicable exit from Daisy, wrists first, which was lymphoma-unrelated). And I was genuinely terrified.

"I'm in trouble."

"Not necessarily," he replied. "We think you have lymphoma, which is a type of cancer. It's pretty treatable. But I can't be sure without a biopsy. So now you have a choice."

"Go," I said. My fear was morphing into anger.

"We can do a needle biopsy, where we stick a needle into the tumor and extract some cells. That would be my second choice."

"Why?" my mother asked.

"It's not a guarantee that I'll get enough cells to make a diagnosis. I'd rather do a full biopsy tomorrow," he said.

"You mean, cut him open?" my mother asked.

"Yes. I'd like to cut a substantial piece out to make sure we get this right."

## 6: THE TIP OF MY ICEBERG

"Let's do it," I said. I liked this guy's guts. My parents started to protest my decision. It was a fruitless venture.

"I think you're making the right decision, Mr. Duffy. Can you be at the surgery center tomorrow at 5:30?"

"a.m.?"

Dr. Pennell laughed. "Yeah, I know."

"I'll be there."

"Pick up your surgery sheet on the way out. You'll need a couple of things from the drug store," he said.

Later, I cursed his couple of things. One was a bottle of magnesium citrate, or "bowel prep," as they call it. I, un-affectionately, dubbed it *colon blow*.

And the only word that comes close to capturing the essence of the experience is *violent*.

Or *brutal*.

Maybe *unholy*.

And just who do they think they're kidding with the whole lemon-lime flavoring? Sprite, this isn't.

—

"Hello?"

"Steph, it's me."

I had no idea what to say. I was afraid for multiple reasons.

"What did they say?"

Per usual, I delivered the news via blurt. "They think I have lymphoma."

Silence. For a good ten seconds. I heard a faint sniffle in the background.

"Are you okay?" I asked.

"Not really." She tried to manage a laugh. She wasn't successful.

"I…um…I know we haven't been together very long," I ventured, "and…um…I don't expect you to be here for this. But… uh…when it's over, if you're still around, I'd love to take you out again." I meant it with every fiber of my being.

"No. No, no, no. We're going to fight this together." She meant it with every fiber of her being.

We said "I love you" and hung up the phone. I stood in the lobby of the hospital and took a deep breath. My parents sat in a corner, giving me as much privacy as you can get in the lobby of a hospital. I walked over to them.

"How is she?" they asked in unison.

"She's okay."

We looked at each other. Silent. Still. In the lobby of a hospital.

"Guys…I'm going to marry that girl."

—

I was wrapped like a mummy and surrounded by nurses, assistants, and Dr. Pennell.

"You ready?" Dr. Pennell asked.

"Take care of me, doc," I told him.

"I promise you I will."

The anesthesiologist lowered the gas mask over my mouth and nose.

"Count backwards from ten," instructed the nurse.

"Ten…nine…eight…"

# 7

## THREE LITTLE WORDS

Seven days after visiting my local urgent care, I sat in the waiting room of a man who could change my life with a single sentence.

His name was Dr. Burton Needles. How fabulous is that? I wondered if his real name was John Smith and he changed it, like a porn star creates a stage name. After all, who knew that little Alden Brown would grow up to be not-so-little Peter North?

Dr. Needles was an unassuming man, five-foot-seven, one-thirty. He wore glasses and really expensive pants. His tie—which probably cost more than a Yugo—was kept in check by a white lab coat. A stethoscope draped itself around his neck. Dr. Needles had intellectual swagger. He smiled, and I liked him immediately. What I didn't like was that it was already Monday, and Dr. Needles still did not have my test results. My surgery had been three days earlier, on Friday. I mean, how long can it possibly take to grab cells removed from a gargantuan tumor and test them repeatedly while knocking out everything they couldn't be until there is not a shred of possible doubt that the physicians have made the right diagnosis with unequivocal accuracy?

"We should have them by tomorrow, if not later today," he told me. "You're young. You're healthy. That's in your favor."

The thought crossed my mind to inform him that though I may have been young, my favorite dinner was a medium pepperoni, sausage, mushroom, and onion pan pizza from Pizza Hut and a Great Biggie Fries from Wendy's. At one sitting. But then again, I didn't think it would help the situation. I just nodded. Young. Healthy. My favor.

Evening rolled around, and still there was no call from the doctor. I knew I wouldn't be getting any test results that day. I lay on my bed at my parents' house, trying any way to get comfortable. The pain was intolerable now. And it was constant.

Delirious from anguish, I remembered an old movie I had seen on HBO back when MTV played nothing but videos and *The Young Ones* on Sunday nights. It was called *Mask*, and it was the true story of a kid named Rocky Dennis.

Rocky Dennis was a real kid who suffered from a disease called Craniodiaphyseal Dysplasia, or Lionitis. It affects only one in every 220 million births. Calcium build-up in Rocky's skull caused unimaginable headaches, deformities, poor eyesight, and death at the age of sixteen.

During one scene in the movie, Rocky tells his doctor his new method of dealing with the excruciating headaches: he talks to them. By conversing with his headaches, he took away the emotional power that the physical power tried to exert.

So I started talking to my tumor. I called it every four and twelve-letter word in the book. I poked it and waggled my finger at it. I yelled at it. I screamed at it. I called it a bully and a coward, and I told the bastard that it would never beat me. And for a few minutes, the pain subsided a bit.

Of course, it came roaring back with a vengeance. *Think you can take me? I dare you!*

*Just you wait,* I thought. *Just you wait.*

—

"Dan? It's Dr. Needles on the phone."

My mom ran up the stairs two at a time, phone in hand. She handed it to me along with the instructions not to talk to him before she could pick up another phone and listen in. I held the phone close to my body and hummed the *Jeopardy!* theme song yet again.

"Okay, Danny!" my mom yelled.

"Hello?"

"Dan? It's Dr. Needles."

"Hi, Doctor, how are you?"

"I'm good. In fact, I'm great. We've hit a homerun...it's testicular!" The man was beside himself with joy.

"Testicular?"

"Yes, it's testicular! It's great news!"

"So wait a second. Are you saying I have cancer?"

"Yes, but it's really good news."

"No. You're saying I have cancer."

For the first time, my anger shifted away from my tumor and to the man who would help me kill it. The momentum swing wasn't lost on him. He paused and took a breath. In theory, he thought he was giving me good news. In reality, he was giving me the worst news I'd ever received in my life.

"Yes, Dan. You have cancer. I'm sorry. But I'm also relieved. You have a simple seminoma. Grab a pen."

For the next five minutes, he told me everything I would need to know for the upcoming week. Tomorrow, I would visit him in his office for more blood tests. In two days, a porta-cath would be inserted near my clavicle; this would be the entry point for my cocktail of three chemotherapy drugs. The porta-cath would save my veins from collapsing or even dying. The three drugs were Cisplatin, VP 16, and Bleomycin.

All would be effective.

All would be extremely toxic.

The drugs' side effects would run the gamut: hair loss, nausea (Cisplatin is the number one nausea-causing chemo drug), numbness, mouth sores, potential hearing loss, diarrhea, and extreme fatigue. Just to name a few. He also told me that sterility might be an issue.

The porta-cath would be installed on Thursday. On Friday, I would visit Dr. Needles for the final time before starting treatment.

I hung up the phone and smiled. For the first time in a while, I was surprisingly upbeat.

"Are you alright?" my dad asked, confused.

"I think I've got this," I said. "At least, now I know what it is. And I don't have to be in pain anymore."

And then, stupidly, I did a cartwheel. I hadn't done a cartwheel since grade school. My mom freaked. I landed on my head.

# 8

## FOUR LITTLE WORDS

"Dan, I'm going to admit you."
I'd never seen Dr. Needles look so nervous, and it scared the life out of me. I had hobbled into his office as walking was out of the question; I could barely stand erect. It was as though the tumor knew what was coming, and it was digging in.

"You can't admit me, doc."

"I can't let you walk out of here with the kind of pain you're in."

If he wanted to admit me to the hospital and stick me on a morphine drip, he would have to arrest me to do it.

"I can't. I have plans."

"What plans?"

"I'm asking Stephanie to marry me on Sunday night."

He saw the smile on my face, despite all the suffering. He knew I wasn't bluffing. Taking a deep breath, he smiled back.

"I guess that's a good reason." He walked over and tousled my hair. "Congrats, sir."

"Thanks, man."

We shook hands even though I still couldn't stand up straight.

"Maybe this will help."

He reached into his pocket, pulled out a prescription pad, made a few scribbles, and handed it to me.

"I don't like prescribing this, but under the circumstances…"

I took the sheet of paper. "Oral morphine?"

"Good luck. You're gonna need it."

He smiled and walked out of the examination room.

—

"Hello?"

Stephanie's mom, Michele, had just turned off the vacuum cleaner. I could hear it powering down in the background.

"Hi, Michele. It's Dan."

"Hi, Dan! How are you feeling, honey?"

"I'm good, thank you. Hey, I wanted to ask you how you'd feel about me asking Stephanie to marry me," I blurted.

There was a moment of silence.

"I think that would be wonderful."

"Really?"

"Well, what did you think I'd say?" Michele laughed.

"I didn't know…I've never done this!" I was laughing, too. "Is Dan there, by chance?"

"He's at work. Let me get you his number."

I said goodbye to Michele, hung up, and began to dial the number of the CVS where Dan was a pharmacist. Like father, like daughter. Halfway through dialing, I hung up. It was one thing to call Michele. It felt like quite another to ask a six-foot-five hulk of a man for his daughter's hand in marriage.

I started dialing again…and hung up. Why was this so hard? What's he going to say? He loves me!

I gave myself an impressive pep talk before dialing the number a third time. It rang once before I hung up.

Taking a deep breath, I stood up, almost fell down, steadied myself, and hobbled around the room, trying to think of something to say, a soliloquy of such elegance that my words alone would beat his cold heart into submission.

*Dan is one of the most warm-hearted guys I know,* I told myself. *Don't be an idiot.*

I dialed a final time.

"Hello, and thank you for calling CVS Pharmacy," the answering system greeted me. "Did you know that you can have your prescriptions renewed automatically?"

No, actually, I didn't know that.

"Just ask your CVS pharmacist today!"

I would try to remember this for later.

"For health and beauty, press one. For liquor, press two. To ask the pharmacist for his daughter's hand in marriage, press three."

The oral morphine had just kicked in.

I pressed three. And I hummed the *Jeopardy!* theme-song.

"CVS, this is Dan."

"Hi, Dan. It's Dan Duffy."

"Well, hello, sir, how are you feeling?"

"I'm good, thanks."

"That's good!"

The small talk was getting us nowhere.

"Dan, I just want you to know that I love your daughter very much, and I would like your permission to ask her to marry me."

And there was silence on the other end of the line. Why is there always silence?

"Dan, you've made me so happy," Steph's dad misted. "Yes, you have my blessing."

—

I arrived at Richard's house at 2:00 p.m. that Sunday. I told Stephanie he needed me to help him move a couch, to which she replied, "Doesn't that jacksauce know what kind of pain you're in?"

In reality, Richard had agreed to host an engagement party for us that night, a night I had planned to perfection.

At 5:50 p.m., I would pick up Stephanie to take her to dinner.

At 6:00 p.m., we would arrive at the Ritz Carlton, where we would be escorted to a corner booth in their fantastic restaurant, The Grill. We would dine on filet and vegetables and chocolate soufflé for dessert. We would drink wine and laugh and talk about the future.

At 8:00 p.m., we would leave the Ritz, and I would drive her to the same rooftop parking lot where I told her I was not leaving for Los Angeles. We would continue to talk about the future. Or dinner. Or the weather. Or "Jacksauce" Richard and his now-moved couch.

## 8: FOUR LITTLE WORDS

At 8:15 p.m., I would pop the question. I had Michele's permission. I had Dan's blessing. I had an engagement party arranged in secret, arranged under the alibi of moving a couch. For a jacksauce. At 8:30 p.m., we would arrive at Richard's house, where my parents, our friends, and our loved ones would be waiting for us to celebrate.

What could possibly go wrong?

I stopped by the grocery store to pick up some cleaning supplies on my way to Richard's. As I scrubbed the toilet on my hands and knees, I told him of my master plan.

"But dude," he asked, "what if she says no?"

"Uhh…" I stammered. "Shut up."

I grabbed some Tidy Bowl out of the shopping bag and was about to attach it on the inside of the toilet tank when Richard stopped me.

"Can't use that shit. It's Hutch's water bowl."

"You let your dog drink out of the toilet?"

"Why do you think it's so clean?"

"You swine."

―

Stephanie excused herself to use the powder room. We were at The Grill at the Ritz Carlton. I reached into the inner pocket of my jacket. The ring was still there. *Of course the ring is still there. Where the hell else would it be?*

I'd been inadvertently playing with the box throughout the entire dinner. I'm sure Steph was wondering why I kept rubbing my left nipple.

The week prior, my parents and my friend Meredith, whom we affectionately call Muzz, went with me to Michael Genovese Jewelers to help me pick the perfect ring.

Picking out a diamond is quite the feat. I knew I wanted something elegant and classic. My idea was one large diamond on a six-pronged platinum band, which met the approval of everyone. I tossed my budget on the table, and Joe Genovese brought out approximately twenty diamonds. We whittled the selection down to two.

One was one-point-nine carats and a hair's breath away from flawless. It was, quite simply, stunning. The other was two-point-zero-one carats and dazzling in every way. But I'm a Virgo and thus a perfectionist. My thought was to pick the more perfect diamond, even though it was slightly smaller.

"Get the two," Muzz said. She was adamant. "Her girlfriends will ask the size, and it'll make a big difference is she can say, 'It's over two carats' instead of 'It's almost two carats.' Trust me."

My mom agreed. "They're both lovely, but the two carat is… wow."

My dad could not have cared less. "You could get her a nice cubic zirconia."

I laughed. Marie and Muzz were not amused.

"You are such a child," my mother said. "Don't listen to him, Danny."

So I picked the two. Peer pressure.

Now a week later, just a day before quite possibly the most important moment of my life, I questioned every facet of my choice. *Did I pick the right diamond? Was it really as pretty as I thought it was?*

As I paced a groove in the carpet through the middle of the store, waiting for the ring to be retrieved from the safe, I heard—faintly—a song playing through a small speaker in the ceiling. It was a song close to Stephanie and me, and it was the first time I'd heard it in any forum besides my own CD player.

In the mid-1980s, Elton John released an epic live album from Australia. It spawned the worldwide re-dominance of one of his old classics, *Candle in the Wind*. However, on the same album, there is a very short, very obscure, but very beautiful song called, *I Need You To Turn To*.

I'm a huge Elton John fan. I think he's one of the greatest songwriters in history. But of all his songs, this song, one of his simplest, speaks to me the most. When Steph and I first started dating, I played the song for her on my car's enormous sound system. She said it was one of the prettiest songs she'd ever heard. And, as a Christmas present, I had the words of the chorus printed on a really nice fabric paper and got it framed.

And here I found myself singing to this very faint, very obscure, very beautiful song in the middle of Michael Genovese Jewelers. I took it as a sign. At that point, however, I probably would have interpreted hitting every green light on the way home as a sign: *God wants me to get home quickly so I can ask her to marry me!* Hell, it wouldn't even have taken that much. I remember sitting on the toilet, playing *Pocket Yahtzee!* and thinking, *If I score over 225, she's going to accept my proposal!* And then I'd roll 206.

*Double-or-nothing!*

"I love the view up here."

Leaning against the four-foot wall near the front my car, Steph and I gazed up at the stars. The sky was late-winter clear, but the night was warm enough to remind us that spring was around the corner.

We were at our parking lot in Clayton, the same parking lot where I told her I wouldn't leave her for Los Angeles. Below, we could hear revelers celebrating St. Patrick's Day. Even though it was a Sunday, the din was impressive. We giggled at the sound of someone vomiting in the distance.

Stephanie must have thought that I was looking for one last little moment of respite before heading home to face chemotherapy in the morning for the first time. She would have been wrong.

My knees figuratively and literally knocked. All I could think was, *Dude, what if she says no?*

*Thank you, Richard. Thank you, 206 in* Pocket Yahtzee!

I swallowed hard. "I have a wild story to tell you."

I walked to the ajar passenger door of my car and ejected the mix CD from my car stereo, replacing it with Elton John.

"What's the story, morning glory?" She was happy from the view. And from the exceptional bottle of wine we had ordered with dinner.

"So I was in a store yesterday, and for the first time ever, I heard this song." I pressed play on *I Need You To Turn To*.

"Oh, I love that song," she smiled.

I walked back to her and took her hands. We danced for the first minute of the three-minute song. It was now or never. I backed up.

"So the store I was in…was Michael Genovese Jewelers. And the song was playing while I was waiting for this…"

# 8: FOUR LITTLE WORDS

I plucked the box from the inside pocket of my jacket. She covered her mouth with her hands. Slowly, I lowered myself to one knee. *Ugh. Pain.* My back didn't care that I was about to propose.

"I knew from the first night I met you, as I had to beat the lesbians off of you, that I wanted to spend forever with you."

Her shoulders shook as she laughed, not making a sound, her mouth still covered. Then, unexpectedly, she dropped to one knee, too. There we were, knee to knee. I continued.

"You are still with me, even after all we've been through in such a short time. I want to spend forever making you as happy as you make me."

My back was giving out. My romantic genuflection capsized to a kneel.

"I love you more than anyone or anything I've ever loved in my life."

Her romantic genuflection capsized to a kneel, though not because of her back. I opened the box. Her eyes popped and welled with tears. There we were, kneeling in front of each other. She happily sobbed. The moment got to me as well, as did my now-fully seized lower back.

"Will you marry me?"

"Oh, my God! Yes!" *In your face, Richard. And* Pocket Yahtzee!

We smashed our faces together and kissed. We may have even smacked teeth together. After a few seconds, we stopped and smiled, like two Cheshire cats.

"I think I need to stand up," I said. "And you might have to help me."

My vertebrae were toast.

Stephanie took my hand and helped me up. I took the ring out of the box and gently slid it onto her finger.

"Wow! It's perfect! How did you know my size?"

*Because I'm good.*

A month prior, my parents had taken Steph and me to see *Phantom of the Opera* at the historic Fox Theater in St. Louis. That night, she just happened to be wearing a ring her grandmother had given her. It was a very intricate piece of jewelry, and I asked if I could see it. She took it off her ring finger and handed it to me. As luck would have it, the ring fit perfectly on my left pinky. When Joe Genovese asked me Stephanie's ring size, I held out my far left digit.

"It's this, exactly."

—

I remember Stephanie calling her parents from my car to tell them the news. I remember being hugged by my own parents at Richard's house. I remember a room full of friends and love and lots of hugging. I remember my brother, Gavin, giving me a pep talk about the next day's chemo treatment, my first. I remember hearing Richard's dog, Hutch, barking up from the basement. *Is that food I smell? I know I smell food! Why am I down here, alone? You all suck.*

But that is about all I can recall, as I have only fragments of memories from that evening. I tried to focus, to comprehend everything that was going on, but I was in a physical and emotional daze.

Two hours after I dropped my fiancé off at her apartment, I wrestled with the beast in a battle for my sanity. My tumor, my bully, tried to murder me using nothing more than horrific pain. There was no relief. I couldn't stand. I couldn't sit. I couldn't lie down. The sheets had long left the bed. The oral morphine was as

## 8: FOUR LITTLE WORDS

useful as an ashtray on a Harley. I found a jar of thick blue cream called Super Blue Stuff. It promised fast, effective relief through its super powerful *emu oil*.

It lied.

Pain makes you think interesting things. As I slathered liquid Smurf guts all over myself, I felt bad for the emus. *How do you oil an emu?* I thought. *It can't be pretty. It can't feel good. Poor emus.* By that point, I was legitimately out of my mind. If Smurf guts helped lessen my pain, I would have happily Smurfed every Smurfy one of them with a big, Smurfy brick.

I was a giant, agitated ball of kinetic energy.

"Get your licks in now," I screamed at my tumor. "Get them in now, do you hear me? Get them in. Kill me if you can, because tomorrow, you are so fucking dead. Do you hear me? Fucking dead!"

A few seconds later, slathered in a blanket of Smurf tragedy, I lost consciousness.

# 9

# MY SECOND GREAT EMBARRASSMENT

"**Mr. Duffy?**"
The nurse at the Washington University Infertility and Reproductive Medicine Center had a face as caring as a child with a mouth full of Sour Patch Kids. She looked like she'd already had a bad day. It was 9:14 a.m.

There are times in my life when I work like an elephant. There are other times when I am procrastination's Gemini. On this occasion, I had put myself squarely behind the eight ball.

It was Monday, March 18, 2002, and, according to the *Kick Cancer's Ass* plan, it was my first day of chemotherapy. Had I followed Dr. Needles's instructions when I was supposed to have followed them, I would have already been in the middle of my first infusion. Instead, I was playing catch-up at the spank bank.

"Do you want to have children?" Dr. Needles had asked five days earlier.

"With you?"

"No, you goof. Do you plan on having children?"

Honestly, I had never thought about it.

"I don't know," I stumbled. "I guess. Maybe? I'm not sure."

"But it's not something that you would completely rule out," Dr. Needles clarified.

"Oh, no. I'd never rule it out."

"Then I suggest you make some fertility plans."

The phrase "fertility plans" meant that the cocktail of chemotherapy drugs I was about to receive boasted an impressive success rate murdering swimmers. Thus, before the assault, I needed to make a *deposit* at the *bank*.

"I'll take care of it," I said.

"Taking care of it" meant that by Monday morning, I had yet to seal the deal. The only thing I could do was visit the fertility clinic, tickle the puppet, and head to the infusion center afterwards.

"Coming," I said to the nurse. "No pun intended."

She pretended not to hear me, but I knew better.

She led me through a sterile white hallway in her sterile white uniform holding a cup that looked to be quite sterile. My mind was swimming with what potentially lay behind door number four. *A stripper pole? Video? A bed with rubber cheetah-pattern sheets?*

Wrong, wrong, and wrong. As the door opened, I was led into a room with four white walls, a hard couch covered in white paper,

## 9: MY SECOND GREAT EMBARRASSMENT

and an old wood grain chest of drawers which was filled with what my friend Subash would call "sub-optimal filth."

*This is it? Are they kidding?*

"Now," Nurse Ratchet continued, "here are the rules. You are to manually bring yourself to climax where you will deposit your semen in this cup."

As she held it, I pictured one of Barker's Beauties from *The Price Is Right* showcasing it with flowing hands during the Mountain Climber game. The yodeling song popped into my head. For approximately a half second.

"Mr. Duffy, are you listening?"

"Yes. Hit in the cup."

If looks could kill…

"You are not allowed to open the cup until right before climax because of the possibility of contaminating the inside of the cup."

Wasn't I already going to contaminate the inside of the cup?

"When you release your ejaculate, make sure that your penis does not touch the inside of the cup for the possibility of contaminating the specimen."

It all sounded so sexy.

"And before you clean up, you must put the top back on the cup immediately and deposit the cup in the receptacle on the wall."

"Anything else?" I asked.

"No. I will be at the front desk when you are finished."

And with that, she walked out of my life. *(tither.)*

As soon as the door closed behind her, I dropped my jeans and boxers to the floor, but prudently kept my shirt on. I looked at the cup in all its sterile wonder. *I'll be out of here in ten minutes*, I thought.

Ha. That notion fled the moment I opened up the top drawer.

"Playboy? Seriously?"

Now don't get me wrong, Playboy has some great articles; but on the porn scale, they rank about as high as an earthworm.

"Next."

The smut factor of the next few magazines wasn't much better. For starters, it was all guy-girl, most of it missionary position. No lesbians. No threesomes. No sixty-nine. And honestly, no landscaping. One lady looked like she had Will Ferrell in a scissor-lock.

"This is bullshit!"

I was irritated, even more so when I looked at my watch and saw that I had been in the room for eight minutes and had yet to manage a single tug.

I brought the least sucky magazine over to the couch. *I bet this thing has more ass juice than a Huggies convention*, I thought as I sat down. Thank God for the tissue paper.

I opened the magazine to the only decent picture available to me. After one minute, I knew I had picked the wrong magazine. I walked back to the chest, found a few more, and sat back down on the couch for another crack.

I flipped magazine pages with my left hand while my right hand stayed "busy." None of the pictures were doing anything for me. I decided to switch hands. A friend had once told me, "If you use your non-dominant hand, it feels like someone else is doing it."

That friend is an idiot. It made no difference. I looked at my watch. Seventeen minutes. Nothing to show for it. *This is going nowhere.*

I tossed the magazines on the floor and lay down on my back on the couch, which, I realize in hindsight, probably wasn't the most comfortable or sanitary position. I tried erasing everything from my mind but Stephanie. We had been together only a few

## 9: MY SECOND GREAT EMBARRASSMENT

months, and as tremendously hot as she is, we didn't have the vast wealth of experience that I really could have used at that moment.

I thought of us in various stages of *rowr* and, for a minute, it looked like it would work. There was a definite surge of adrenaline with a particular thought, and I worked myself over like a toddler molding Play-Doh.

And then, I hit the wall—the wall being the thought *What if this doesn't happen?* I struggled to pull my thoughts back to each immaculate curve of Stephanie's body. Instead, I was trapped under the shroud of *What if I can't finish? If I can't do this, and then I get chemo, are my chances over forever?*

And with that, twenty-four minutes of struggle ended in defeat. I had failed. And all I had to show for my efforts was an empty cup and a small rug burn. It was the second greatest embarrassment of my life.

I won't tell you the first, except to say that it involved a fancy hotel and a loss of bodily function. And before you ask, I was sober.

Dejection turned to irritation. Irritation turned to fear. I realized I might never be able to have children. Blackness descended over my heart and my soul. I had failed myself. I had failed Stephanie. I had failed any children I might have had.

I got dressed and walked out of the room, empty cup in hand. At the desk, Nurse Ratchet looked at my lifeless eyes and then at the cup.

"Do it at home. Same rules as before. Get it back to us within a half hour of completion." And then, in a moment of utter humanity, she added, "It happens more than you think."

When growing up in my house, I tried every trick in the book to hide my masturbatory practices. Running the faucets, locking the bathroom door, coughing loudly, and fifty-three minute showers were my preferred methods. It was quite another matter now that my parents knew what was going on, and worse, encouraged it.

"Good luck," said my dad. Probably didn't need to hear that.

After downloading every naughty pic I could find, I finally hit the lottery with two girls and a number. Of course, at the moment of truth, having to pull off more maneuvers than a juggling clown to not mess up my chances made me wholly dissatisfied with the entire affair.

I closed the cup, wrapped it in a towel, got dressed, and had my dad drive me back to see my new girlfriend. She was going to be so proud of me.

I had finally succeeded in my attempt to save any potential lineage, eighteen hours *after* completing my first round of chemotherapy.

# 10

## DODGED THE BULLET (I THOUGHT)

At my appointment on the Wednesday before chemotherapy, Dr. Needles asked my parents and me if we had any questions. My dad, who never says anything to doctors, pulled this out of...*somewhere*.

"Doctor, when my dad died of cancer, I started donating to Sloan Kettering, as kind of a tribute. A few months ago, they sent me a letter thanking me for being a benefactor, and if there was anything they could ever do for me, to let them know. Would you be willing to call them to see if your course is the best course for treating my son?"

My mother and I were floored. So was Dr. Needles. My father hadn't said a word to him since "Nice to meet you" the week before.

The journey up to this point had been a whirlwind. My life hurtled from chronic back pain to chemotherapy in less than fourteen days. In the midst of the tumbling, I never even thought to ask for a second opinion. I mean, had Dr. Needles been a perineum, we might have thought about it. But we loved the guy, and he really seemed to have our best interest at heart.

"Mr. Duffy, I did my residency at Sloan Kettering. I'll be happy to call them."

My mother, my father and I were floored. This man had a brilliant mind and an amazing track record, and he was willing to toss aside any ego he might have had. At that moment, I knew I would trust the man with my life and that I would be okay.

As it turned out—and much to everyone's surprise, including Dr. Needles's— one of my chemotherapy drugs was deemed unnecessary. A few weeks earlier, after extensive research, the folks at Sloan Kettering discovered that for a simple seminoma, the type of cancer I had, Cisplatin and VP-16 would suffice. Bleomycin could be dropped.

When I researched the side effects of Bleomycin, also known as "the carpet bomber," I thought I had dodged a bullet the size of New Jersey. Darkening of the skin, pain, fever, vomiting, weight loss, mouth sores, skin blisters, rash, and hair loss.

*Thank Christ. None of that,* I thought.

And for the first three days of my chemotherapy, I felt only one thing: pain relief. I had been preoccupied with all of the tests and infusion sessions and the poking and prodding. All the hubbub was inconvenient, but it was an excellent distraction from the reason of all the hubbub in the first place: my tumor.

"How is the pain?" my dad asked me after my third infusion. The fact that I had to stop and think about it gave me my answer. I did a few twists and even attempted a few inflexible toe touches.

"Dad? It's gone."

It's amazing what a bit of good news will do for you. Suddenly, I felt like I could take on the world! If my physical condition was any indication, the drugs were working! In just three days! And not only that, but I had yet to experience a single side effect! I *totally* had this!

Every thought I was having ended with an exclamation point! On day three!

*Day Four.* Nausea. Overwhelming, devastating nausea.

There is not a single word that can describe *Day Four*. On *Day Four*, you feel like death, plus hell, plus ass. You are on the verge of physically collapsing at any moment. Your entire body aches. And your stomach is so twitchy that even the slightest movement results in puking up your toenails. For someone who hates vomiting, there is no worse feeling in the world.

Despair eventually trumps your own will, and you realize that your only recourse is make it to the toilet, drop to your knees, hold on to the seat, take a deep breath, and expel everything in your belly.

Of course, at that moment it was 7:00 a.m. The entire contents of my belly consisted of an ounce of water and some bile.

If you've ever vomited like this, usually after a bender or a bout of food poisoning, you know that the taste alone elicits retching, making you gag and try to throw up even more. But there's nothing left to throw up, and now your already twitchy belly goes into muscle spasms so fierce that you recoil into the fetal position in self-defense.

You breathe hard, first through your nose and eventually through your mouth, because you simply can't get enough air through your nostrils. After a couple of minutes, your muscles relax, and you move from your knees to your butt, slumped against the wall, praying that you never again have to suffer through such a horrendous experience. My only silver lining was that I was able to maintain control of other…orifices…while doing what I could to survive this ordeal. All of the training in my early twenties had finally paid off.

"God, if you get me out of this," you pray, pleading for it to be over.

But there's a really ugly secret with chemo puking: after you have thrown up, you don't feel any better. At all. In fact, you feel worse, because once you realize that throwing up doesn't help, you fear it. Each episode is so brutal that you will do anything you can to keep from participating again. You move slower. You avoid food, partly because you know you won't keep it down, partly because nothing sounds good. For nutrition, you drink things like Ensure, Gatorade, and Pedialyte, because God help you if you dehydrate.

All of this happens the first day the nausea hits. And it only gets worse. Being violently ill is bad enough without the caveat that you literally have no idea if or when it will end.

Days after finishing my first cycle of chemo, I was still sick. And in the spirit of the *American Top 40*, the hits just kept on coming. Eight mornings after my first infusion, and in the midst of my vomitorious purgatory, my head felt "itchy." I opened my eyes and scratched my scalp with both hands. When I brought them down in front of my face, it looked like I brought a gorilla to climax.

"Oh, shit."

The bullet must have missed me on the first pass, but apparently it circled back and hit me square in the head, knocking my ego to the floor. Or, the drain, to be exact. A quick shower two minutes later revealed I'd lost enough hair to craft at least a half-dozen quality merkins. Any confidence of keeping my hair that I'd enjoyed had shattered into a pile of three-inch red strands collecting in the drain of my bathtub.

I had promised myself that I would not let cancer take my hair. I swore I wouldn't give it that type of power. I'd take it myself before I let cancer take it, dammit. In other words, "If you don't play how I want to play, I'm taking my ball and going home."

At the time, it seemed perfectly logical.

I headed to the kitchen of my parents' house. My mom was waiting for me.

"It's falling out," I said. "I'm getting it shaved."

"It doesn't look like it's falling out," she tried to comfort me.

I put my right index finger and thumb against my scalp and plucked a fresh tuft of hair. *Exhibit A*. I walked over to the trash compactor and was about to eliminate the evidence, but my mother told me just to leave it in the counter. She would take care of it.

What I didn't know was that as soon as I walked out the door, she raced upstairs and collected every last hair she could find. She has them in an envelope to this day.

—

"You're coming with me to the Super Snips. We're shaving it."

I stood in the doorway of Richard's front room, the same room where we celebrated my engagement nine days prior. He was sitting on the alibi couch.

"Bullshit."

Richard jumped up, ran his hand through my hair, and pulled out a fistful.

"Satisfied?"

"Holy crap, that's the coolest thing I've ever seen!" He was beside himself with an odd glee.

"Thanks for that, ass."

"I know just the chick."

---

I could not stop looking at my reflection in the rearview mirror. For the first time since I was in utero, I was hairless. I didn't quite know what to think. Thankfully, I didn't have any warts or excessive moles. My melon wasn't pointy. And, surprisingly, I really didn't look all that sick. I just looked bald. It wasn't a bad thing. It wasn't a good thing. It was just…a thing.

Richard called our friend Chris and asked if he wanted to join us for lunch. A few minutes later, as we pulled into Chris' driveway, I asked Richard not to make a big deal out of it in front of him.

"I just don't want him to feel self-conscious, like he has to say something or treat me with kid gloves."

"I get it."

"It's just that…people are going to treat me differently. I don't want that. I don't want anyone to feel uncomfortable. I'm just…me. Okay?"

"You're good enough…you're smart enough…"

## 10: DODGED THE BULLET (I THOUGHT)

"Shut it."

I threw the car in park. Richard reached over and honked the horn a dozen times. The man has the tact of a bull shark. Chris opened the front door of his house and walked out.

"Not a word," I muttered to Richard.

Chris opened the back door of my car and climbed in. He closed the door and put his seatbelt on. Once it clicked, he looked me in the eye, stared at my head for a few seconds, and finally spoke.

"Ya know," he said, trying to find the words, "you kinda look like the tip of my dick."

# 11

## MAY OR MAY NOT CAUSE BONE PAIN

In his 1933 inaugural address, President Franklin D. Roosevelt uttered the immortal phrase, "The only thing we have to fear is fear itself." We all know the first part of the quote, but almost more important is the second: "…nameless, unreasoning, unjustified terror which paralyzes needed efforts to convert retreat into advance."

As humans, when we are faced with any kind of tragedy or crisis, one of the first things we do is personalize it. It helps to make the intangible tangible; to make the unknown known; to make the strange less foreign.

I learned quickly that cancer was going to hit me like a truck. The only control I had was in the choice to brace for impact or be run over. School House Rocky told me early in my childhood, "Knowledge is Power!" Little bastard was right.

I spent quite a bit of time researching my disease on the internet. Testicular cancer first appeared in the public consciousness through a movie called *Brian's Song*. It tells the true story of Brian Piccolo, a member of the Chicago Bears who is diagnosed with the disease. The film also illustrates Piccolo's friendship with his teammate Gayle Sayers as he battles through illness and treatment. Piccolo died on June 16, 1970. He was twenty-six.

Then, in 1974, a doctor named Lawrence Einhorn began studying an experimental drug called Cisplatin and its effects on testicular cancer cells. The trial, which was a Phase II study, was so outrageously successful that Phase III was deemed medically unnecessary. Cisplatin became the gold standard in the treatment of the disease, turning a killer into something that could be killed.

If the name sounds familiar, Dr. Einhorn is the man who cured cyclist—and Livestrong founder—Lance Armstrong of testicular, lung, and brain cancer. That doc is a badass.

I became fairly learned in the potential side effects of the drugs I was taking. Some were already in full swing; some had yet to show up. Sweating and puking? Check. Mouth sores and rash? Negative.

By far, the most painful of these effects was the sneaky bonus of constipation. Constipation is not high on the list of potential ailments. In fact, diarrhea is far more common. But what bothered me the most was how long it took me to realize it was happening.

At the peak of my first waltz with nausea, I stopped eating. Nothing sounded good, not even bananas. (A banana, I must note, is the only food that tastes the exact same way going down as it does coming up.) I chalked up my lack of appetite to queasiness. I couldn't force myself to eat (much to the chagrin and fear of my mother).

What I hadn't considered was the possibility of another, more devious side effect causing my discomfort. It wasn't that I simply didn't *want* to eat. I literally *couldn't* eat. After a week of retching, I started to have the occasional desire for food. Yet, after two or three bites, I'd have to stop. At first, I couldn't figure out why. Until one day, when I suffered a burp that tasted like a fart.

My insides had totally and completely shut down. Digestion had ceased. I couldn't eat because there was no room left for… anything. The garbage pile of undigested food serpentined from the middle of my esophagus to the very end of my large intestine where the clog began. Week-old chicken remnants were rotting inside of me, and I was unable to do anything about it.

I counted backwards to the last time I remembered pooping. Twelve days. *Twelve days?* I called Dr. Needles's office in panic.

"Okay, this is gonna sound gross," I told Valerie, Dr. Needles's administrative assistant, "but I can't poop."

After her muffled phone laughter subsided, Valerie put me through to the nurse who in turn suggested Metamucil and a stool softener.

"What about magnesium citrate?" I asked.

"That would be unsafe," she responded.

The word "unsafe" sounded *unsafe*. Stool softener it was.

It took three agonizing days for the stool softener to soften the stool. But once it did…sweet Mother of Jesus.

Very few times in my life have I had the pleasure of enjoying "Wisdom Teeth Pain." I coined the phrase when I was twenty-two and had to have all four wisdom teeth removed at once. The top were a snap. The bottom two had to be hacked out of my jaw. When the first round of pain meds wore off, I started doing sit-ups in bed, screaming my life out.

Fast-forward seven years to the post-apocalyptic dumping ground bred by several doses of stool softener and two weeks of backlog. If the nurse was shooting for excruciating, she overshot it by several miles. The whole experience reminded me of an old joke:

"In a public restroom, how do you know the person before you was constipated?"

"Teeth marks in the door."

As I attempted to defile my bathroom for the first time in almost a fortnight, I yanked the bath towel off the bar in front of me and bit right through it. Seriously. I held one end of the towel in each hand as I flailed in anguish and bit down so hard that the "Thick & Thirsty" ripped right in two.

And that was just the first bout. I had yet to pass the vast majority of putrefaction still lodged in my gut, an event, which, I regret to report, happened several days later at a Chinese restaurant, obliging me to leave a hundred-dollar tip for damages.

But as much as the constipation blindsided me, the side effect that surprised me the most was the one I didn't even understand in the first place: leucopenia, otherwise known as low white blood cell count. And this one, by far, was the most dangerous.

Chemotherapy is great at killing a lot of things. Specifically, it's great at killing rapidly dividing cells, like cancer cells, hair cells, the cells of your stomach lining, and white blood cells.

Yes, those white blood cells, the ones which fight off infection.

## 11: MAY OR MAY NOT CAUSE BONE PAIN

The Monday after my inaugural round of infusions, I continued on my quest to endure enough blood tests to make my arm look like that of a heroin addict.

"Dan, your white blood cell count is low," Dr. Needles informed me.

"How low?"

"Zero."

"Excuse me?"

At that moment, my body had absolutely no defense in fighting off an infection. On the upside, cold and flu season was over! On the downside, I had no white blood cells!

Dr. Needles explained that despite its gravity, leucopenia was only a minor setback. We would start a course to build them back up. That course would require two thousand dollars' worth of shots (Thank you, insurance!), and those shots would be self-injected.

"But don't worry," Dr. Needles assured me. "The nurses across the hall will help you with the first couple of shots until you're ready to administer them to yourself at home. It will be much easier on you."

Sure it would.

—

"This is Neupogen, and this may hurt."

The nurse plunged a small needle into the top of my thigh.

"We do it here because we need some meat, and it would be hard to give yourself a shot in the posterior."

"What do I worry about with these?" I asked.

"The most common side effect is a burning sensation, so when you do this at home, inject it as slowly as you can. Apart from that, lethargy and possible bone pain."

"Possible?"

"You may not have it."

"Really?"

"But then again, you might."

"What? Which one is it?"

"I don't know."

She was taking great delight in my terror. I was ticked, but her playful wink talked me off the ledge.

—

"You really want to see this?"

"Please."

Stephanie had asked if she could witness my first home self-injection of Neupogen. She was motivated partly by the desire to make sure I was okay and partly by sheer curiosity.

"Okay."

On the first day, the nurse gave me the injection. On the second day, I injected myself in front of her and passed her test with flying colors. And, frankly, it wasn't horrendous. This was my third shot of Neupogen. I had yet to enjoy the bone pain, but I thought better of assuming I'd dodged a…well…you know. I'd been burned by that one before.

I retrieved the syringe from the baggie and removed the safety cover from the needle. Then slowly—methodically—I pierced the skin, pushing the needle into the top of my thigh, near the other

## 11: MAY OR MAY NOT CAUSE BONE PAIN

two needle marks. *How do drugs addicts or people with diabetes do this to themselves?* I wondered.

It took two minutes to push the plunger down approximately one inch. I had an extraordinary fear of the burning sensation I'd been told about, so I did everything I could to avoid it.

When I plucked the needle from my leg, I looked up at Stephanie. She had tears in her eyes.

"I never want to see that again."

It was the first time that she saw me as someone who was sick. She was not prepared.

# 12

## HOLD ME

If I had to get cancer, I got it at the best time imaginable. As divine providence would dictate, I was diagnosed during the only time in my adult life when I happened to be living with my parents. I often look back on those days and marvel at just how blessed and lucky I was.

At twenty-nine years old, even after being thrown out of a flipping Jeep at sixty miles-per-hour, I never gave a whole lot of thought to my mortality. As far as I was concerned, I would live forever. Yet when I heard the words, "You have cancer," the old, eternally insouciant me died. I felt my illusions expire. It was an unexpected demise.

Up to that point, I had been relatively insulated from death. All my close relatives still lived in Ireland when they passed. I was thirty-nine before I attended a funeral that rocked my core.

Now, for the first time in my life, I stared death in the face. And I could do it any time I felt like it; all I had to do was look in the mirror.

If I didn't get any treatment, cancer would kill me, sooner rather than later. Nothing felt secure. Every fortification I had built around my life collapsed. My appetite was gone. My hair was gone. My white blood cells were gone. My normal was gone, and I didn't know how to get it back, if that was even possible. The only thing that was certain was that I wanted to live, and I would do whatever was necessary to survive.

"Dan, we need to cut out a piece of your tumor."

*Done.*

"Dan, you're going to need twenty rounds of poison injections..."

*Great.*

"...through a rubber port we're going to surgically install near your neck..."

*Wonderful.*

"...and each infusion is going to take four hours a day."

*Fantastic.*

"And the cumulative effects you'll suffer will make you want to quit, but you can't quit."

*I'll never quit.*

I once read an amazing blog about what a cancer patient *really* felt going through hell. He talked about how people thought he was so brave in his fight—and how wrong those people were. The blog was dead on.

If you were to poll one hundred cancer patients, chances are not a single one of them would consider himself or herself brave. Personally, I was *terrified* on more occasions than I can count.

Want to hear how brave I was? During my treatment, I sustained literally hundreds of needle pricks in my arms. Not *once* did I look at the needle going in or at my blood going out. I couldn't, all because of that one time in high school when I decided I'd rather donate blood than go to class.

My blood is special—or so I like to think. It's Type O negative, which is universal red cell donor's blood. If you've ever seen one of the countless medical shows on TV, you've heard a doctor or nurse or EMT scream, "We need two units of O-neg, stat!" Almost any patient in need can receive O-neg blood. The Red Cross salivates over O-neg donors.

Never a big fan of high school, I salivated at the thought of any reason to skip class. When the Red Cross stopped by, offering cookies, orange juice, and Domino's Pizza to anyone who donated blood, I jumped at the opportunity. Dodge pre-calculus? Oh hell, yes!

Without a care in the world, I lay down on the cot in the De Smet Jesuit High School gymnasium, home of the Spartans. As the needle sunk into my skin, I thought about the poor schmoes stuck in Mr. Gummels's pre-cal emporium. I chuckled as I looked over at the bag slowly filling with my blood.

What happened next is still a bit of a blur. I was told the whole scene resembled a great Shakespearian tragedy. Or comedy. Or both. Allegedly, I screamed, "Oh, dear God!" before tumbling off the cot and losing consciousness. That was the day I learned I am terrified at the sight of my own blood.

"But Dan," people might say, "even though you winced at the sight of your own blood, you still provided vial after vial of your life force to aid the doctors who were helping you to survive. You are so brave and honorable and sexy."

That bravery was, in reality, resignation. It took a good few days and a lot of convincing from my medical team before I conceded that I was not, in fact, in control. Of anything.

One of the hardest things in the world is to admit you are powerless over your situation. I fought it every step of the way, not wanting to give up yet another illusion of normalcy.

My parents had repeatedly offered to drive me to my chemotherapy infusions—all of them, in fact. Every time they asked, I balked.

"I'm capable of driving myself."

This turned into, "Okay, you can take me to the first one."

Which became, "I guess it would be okay, but just for the first few rounds."

And eventually, "I'd love for you to take me to every infusion. It would make me feel better."

The metamorphosis comes naturally once you let go. It's freeing, even liberating, to be able to say, "I can't do this alone. I'm scared. Hold me and tell me it's going to be okay. Be brave with me. Be brave *for* me, since you, of all people, know how I really feel."

Countless times after my chemo treatments, my mom would sit at the edge of my bed and put her hand on my bald, sweaty head. I can't tell you how good it felt to be cared for.

Sometimes you just want to be loved, and I was. I knew it. I relished it. I embraced it. It allowed me to be a son. It allowed my parents to be parents. And once I was free to love and be loved, it changed everything for the better, and it made the unknown far less frightening.

*The only thing we have to fear is…*

The virtual sanctuary created by my family and Stephanie was a protective shield that I took with me everywhere I went, especially to the infusion center—a traumatic stomping ground in and of itself.

On my first day at "Club Chemo," I had no idea what to expect. My dad sensed my anxiety and asked if he could sit with me during the infusion. Happy for the company, I agreed.

The infusion lab was a sterile rectangle twenty feet wide and sixty feet long with white walls, white tile floors, and a collection of polyurethane recliners in colors that a Glidden paint factory couldn't replicate. In the center of the room was a well-fortified bastion of nurses, monitors, and chemotherapy drugs. The recliners circled this enclosure, giving the impression the nurses were under siege. Each recliner was equipped with a curtain, which could be closed for privacy, and an I.V. pole on wheels, complete with a battery backup. That way, if you had to use the bathroom, you could unplug the pole from the wall and scuttle away.

At first, I was so glad for my dad's company. We chatted for a few minutes, and then, when we ran out of small talk, I broke out a little handheld video game I had purchased for the long treatments. When I got bored with the game, I read a magazine. After that, I checked my watch. Forty-two minutes. I had another three-fifteen to kill. *Shit.*

I thought a game of *Guess the Malady* might be interesting. I glanced around the room without staring, trying to see those with whom I was doing time. There was a young cowboy, my age.

*Possible lymphoma.*

There were a few people in their forties, mostly women, mostly wearing bandanas.

*Breast.*

And then there were what I silently deemed "the Old Guards." The minimum age of the Old Guards was seventy. An Old Guard always had a buddy. Sometimes the buddy was a friend. More often than not, the buddy was a spouse.

*Not a clue, but I'll bet the lady on oxygen has lung.*

I expected something grandiose during that first day, or at least a feeling of wonder or even relief that my tumor was going to be on its last leg soon. Instead, it was more of a subtle, soul-crushing boredom. I tried to meditate; this lasted twelve seconds. I tried to sleep. I used the bathroom twice. I would have killed for a nice long movie. I would have settled for a little TV. Heck, fifteen minutes of Jerry Springer sounded like a dream, even with all the "Have you been hurt in an accident?" commercials.

There was no TV, though. Or music. Or any sound at all besides the IV pole beeping at the patients who forgot to plug them back in after they got back from the bathroom. My dad is a lovely conversationalist, but he is also one of the most introspective men I've ever met, and we sat in a fairly uncomfortable silence. On the surface, he was stoic. I never saw him blink, but I could almost feel the anguish beneath his skin, anguish he tried desperately to subdue.

I still had an hour left in my treatment, and all I could think about was him. I felt so helpless for him. It would be awful to watch your son go through this. How could I reassure him that everything was going to be okay, even when I had no idea if

## 12: HOLD ME

everything was going to be okay? Our hearts were broken that day, each for the other.

I had to do something, and the only way I could imagine surviving this was to play ostrich: if you can't see it, it isn't there.

"Dad, I appreciate you being here more than you know. But I'm worried about you—" how could I put this delicately? —"and at this point, it's not letting me worry about myself. Would you be offended if I asked you just to drive me tomorrow, and then I'll take care of the rest on my own?"

My father, the pillar, took a deep breath. "Dan, I'll do anything you need me to do."

I closed my eyes to keep from tearing up. I was scared to face this on my own, but it's what I thought I had to do.

—

A chemotherapy infusion is a bit like prison. I remember once seeing a convicted felon being interviewed about what it was like being incarcerated, and he said, "The worst thing about it is the time. You have lots of time with nothing but your thoughts."

That line kept echoing in my head repeatedly. I didn't want to think about my situation. I didn't want to face my mortality. The things I did to try blank my mind were just shy of preposterous. Every day, I was infused with two full IV bags of Cisplatin and VP-16. As a little game to focus on something besides my lack of anything fun to do, I would try to *hold it* the entire time, which is no small feat considering I was pumped with a Pepsi two-liter worth of liquid poison. I succeeded only twice. I won't say how many times I *almost* made it. Not my smartest move; I do not recommend doing this.

I always tried to look for the funny with my situation, and most times I could find a nugget or two of the painfully ridiculous that I considered chuckle worthy. This was not the case, however, in the chemotherapy ward. There is nothing fun about sitting in a room surrounded by very real examples of attempted murder by a disease. I tried not to think about it, but I knew that some of these people were not going to make it out of their situation alive.

While the visual was bad, the smell sucked the life out of me. There is no adequate way to describe the odor in the infusion room. It smelled like dying, and it used to hit me from the moment I got off the elevator each morning.

The one thing that got me through most of my days, though, was the commitment of the Old Guards. They were, by far, the highest percentage of the population. They never said much to anyone, even each other. Usually, the patient slept while the spouse kept watch, not daring to avert his eyes from his love or her eyes from her love. I never knew what type of cancer each one had. I never knew if any of them were terminal. I figured it couldn't be easy at their age. It wasn't easy at mine.

But they didn't waver. They didn't falter. They didn't stumble. Their collective quiet, understated power became the stuff of legend in my mind and heart. I often wondered what they thought as they sat their so quietly, staring at nothing in particular. After a while, I started to wonder what if it was me in their situation.

What if, God forbid, Stephanie was diagnosed? Would I ask her to keep fighting, to spend long days—her last days—in a treatment center just to stay alive for me because I would be lost without her? Would I have the strength to understand if she decided to forego treatment because she would have no quality of life? And just say that, God willing, I'm cured, but cancer visits me again

## 12: HOLD ME

later in my life. Would I have the strength to face it again? Would I choose quality over quantity, wanting Steph to see me happy for six months instead of being hooked up to poison for two years? And if it was, indeed, the end, I would want her to be happy. I would tell her that if she found someone else after I died, that it would be okay, as long as he didn't wear any of the clothes she had bought me. And then I pictured her saying that it wouldn't be an issue because Ralph wouldn't fit into my clothes, anyway.

I felt I would go crazy if this was to be my daily routine at the hospital. Tomorrow would be different. Tomorrow, I would find a friend.

—

"Never again."

"What never again?" my dad asked as I climbed into the car.

"I'm never talking to anyone in that place again."

A few hours earlier, he had dropped me off for my infusion. As I got off the elevator, the smell hit me square in the face. I would never get used to it.

I walked into the infusion center. My spot from the day before was occupied. In fact, most of the chairs were occupied. I circled the room before I finally spied a free chair in the corner, right next to the twenty-something cowboy I recognized from my first treatment.

He wore Levi's that were faded from his time in the fields, not from an expensive stonewash. His shirt screamed "Willard" from the original *Footloose*. His wife was by his side; she was pregnant. The whole scene was very Norman Rockwell, if Norman Rockwell had painted *Portrait of a Country Chemo Couple*.

"Mind if I grab this one?" I asked as I moseyed on over to him and sat down, not bothering to wait for an answer. I'm not a moseyer by nature, but thought it appropriate.

"Help yourself, sir."

I offered him my hand.

"I'm Dan."

"Will."

Yes. Seriously.

"What are you in for?" I joked.

He looked from one side of the room to the other before leaning close to me, as though he were about to tell me he'd done something illegal.

"Testicle, sir."

"Ball? Same here."

"Did yours get up in your lymph nodes?" he asked.

"No. Yours?"

"Yes, sir." He hesitated. "That surgery was beyond belief."

He had piqued my curiosity. "Would you tell me about it?"

"Well, they started by cutting me from neck to belly."

I did not like where this was going.

"And once I was open, they took all of my organs out and laid 'em on the table. And then they cut out the lymph nodes and put my organs back in and sewed me back up."

"Holy shit, are you serious?"

I'd never heard anything like that in my life. The doctors got to my cancer before it got to my lymphatic system. I felt a little guilty.

"Yeah. It wiped out our harvest, I'll tell you that."

"That's awful."

"Yeah. And then when the tornado hit…"

I knew I was going to regret it, but I did it anyway.

## 12: HOLD ME

"Tornado?"

"Wiped out the barn. Flipped the tractor, too."

Dear God, it's a country song.

*Twister flipped my tractor...,*

*Cancer took my 'nodes....*

"And now the bank's callin'."

Is this guy asking me for money?

"Don't know what we're gonna do, especially with the little ones on the way."

"Little *ones?*" I asked, fearfully.

"Triplets."

*What?*

"But the good Lord will provide. Somehow." Willard was now almost inconsolable.

I was trapped like a fart in a car. How the hell did I get myself into this? How the hell was I going to get myself out?

"So what do you do for a livin'?" asked Willard.

Opening, here I come.

"I work at Burger King," I lied.

"Do you get free food?"

"Pfft...I wish." I stood up. "Would you excuse me? I have to go throw up. Stupid chemo."

"Oh, I hear, ya," agreed Willard.

And with that, for the first time, I used my cancer to escape a predicament. It would not be the last.

"And then I spent half an hour hiding in the bathroom until Willard finished his treatment and left," I told my dad.

For the first time in a long time, he cackled.

"This shit isn't funny!" I protested.

This sent him into hysterics. I'm glad that Willard's complete and utter tragedy, coupled with my job at Burger King that didn't even come with free food, gave my dad a laugh.

I hadn't heard him laugh in a while. I hadn't realized how much I needed to hear it.

# 13
## THE BEAUTY OF WEEK THREE

"Well, your white count is back up." Dr. Needles seemed pleased with my blood work. "How's the nausea?"
"Been gone for a couple of days."
"Are you eating?"
"Not as much as I'd like him to," said my mom.
"I'm eating fine, thanks." I said.
"And how about bowel movements?"
"We're moving again."
I didn't feel like telling Dr. Needles about the Shrimp Egg Foo Yung—which was amazing, by the way—that had cost me a hundred bucks.

"And what about pain?"

"Gone."

What has two thumbs and could light a room up with his smile? This guy!

"Good, good." Dr. Needles looked over the chart one last time. "Do you have any questions for me? Any side effects?"

"I have a little ringing in my ears every now and then. And sometimes, I sweat like Ted Stryker trying to land a plane."

Dr. Needles laughed. The *Airplane!* reference was not lost on him.

"It's all normal," he said, "but we'll have your hearing tested this week. And I'll set up a CT scan after your next round of treatment."

"Anything I should be doing until then?" I asked.

"Sure. Enjoy week three."

When I first started chemotherapy, I wondered why I had to wait so long between rounds. Couldn't I just do the chemo all at once? Or, at the very least, couldn't we speed things up a bit? Maybe every two weeks?

Once I hit my first week three, it all made sense.

Week one, or infusion week, is a bit like the seventy-two hours before a hurricane. You know the storm is coming, and there's nothing you can do about it.

Week two is hell in all its fury. All you can do is hang on and pray for it to end.

Then comes week three, the calm after the storm. People who have lived through a hurricane often say the sky that comes after the clouds have cleared is such a vivid blue it almost doesn't look real.

Week three is that blue sky.

## 13: THE BEAUTY OF WEEK THREE

Sure, I was surrounded by signs of devastation. I was still gaunt, my appetite was stuck in limbo, and I could have easily been mistaken for Mr. Clean, or at least the spokesperson for Nair. But the nausea had subsided, my energy was restored, and my ability to fight off an infection came roaring back. Cold germs? Come at me, bro. *Come at me!*

Week three is also a psychological watershed. It's the week you learn that if your chemo is working, you've got a fair shot at not dying. Your emotional life changes dramatically with this revelation.

When I first heard the words "you have cancer," I wrapped myself inside the cocoon of family, friends, and fiancé. I wanted to be surrounded by their warmth and laughter and positive energy. I gave up trying to control any situation, placed myself in the hands of others, and in a way, regressed back to my childhood.

Once I thought my chances of survival increased, my courage was buoyed. I wanted to spread my wings a little bit.

Actually, let me rephrase that. Once I thought my chances of survival increased, I attacked liberation like a rabid honey badger that didn't give a shit.

One Sunday, Steph went out with a few friends from Effingham. She asked me if I wanted to go, and I told her that I wasn't feeling it. Maybe the hair loss was getting to me. Maybe I was feeling sorry for myself. Maybe, deep down, I was hoping she'd say, "Oh, Dan, I understand. Why don't I just stay home with you and attend to your every need?"

Instead, I got, "I hope you feel better, and I love you. I'll call you tonight."

As she walked out the door, I realized, yet again, that I was an idiot. I jumped out of bed and took a shower. Showers had become a mixed blessing. Someone once told me that I should shampoo my hairless head to keep the subterranean hair follicles stimulated. I thought it was a crock, but at this point, I wasn't questioning much. I will say, however, that the forty-five second turnover from shower to dressed was a plus.

It really is the little things.

I knew the restaurant where she was meeting her friends, and her look of bewilderment when I showed up unannounced gave me pause. Did she not want me to be there? Was she hiding something? In reality, it was much worse.

"Are you sure you're up for this?" she asked.

"I wouldn't be here if I wasn't," I said without smiling.

When I was first diagnosed with cancer, I worried that people would treat me differently or with kid gloves. In my mind, any kind of changed attitude towards me equaled pity, and I could imagine nothing worse than being pitied.

What I have since learned is that you can't expect humans not to feel human things or not to rely on human emotions. What I interpreted as pity, Stephanie meant as love. When family and friends treated me delicately, it wasn't because they were trying to hurt me; it was because they loved me, and they wanted to do everything in their power to make sure I was okay. And truth be told, I would have done the same thing. In fact, I do. When I see a friend in need, either physically or emotionally, I can't help but jump in with both feet: "What can I do? How can I make this better? Lean on me, when you're not strong. I'll be your friend. I'll help you carry on."

Yes, I actually said that. Once.

I spent the first half an hour at the oyster restaurant regretting being so curt with Stephanie. When we finally had a moment alone, I begged her forgiveness for being a dick.

## 13: THE BEAUTY OF WEEK THREE

"That's fine," she said with zero emotion. It was a brilliant response, because right then, she loved me in the exact way I needed to be loved in that moment. Namely, she kicked my ass for being an ass, cancer or no cancer.

I also learned another valuable lesson that day: I still can't drink tequila. In my younger and stupider days, I had a few knockdown dragouts with one Pepé Lopez, Esquire. He would beat me from pillar to post and then taunt me, daring me to say, "Thank you, sir! May I have another?"

As the day became night and the oyster restaurant became a tiny dive bar with table shuffleboard, Pepé's wealthier, bastard cousin, Patrón, reared his butt-ugly mug. Before I knew it, I barfed up a brussel sprout—and I hadn't eaten one of those in well over a decade.

It occurred to me, as I lay in bed that night, sweating like a Derby horse, that the tequila may not have been my wisest decision. I flung my leg off the bed in a vain attempt to avoid the spins and cursed all things Mexican. The agave nectar. The Taco Bell Cheesy Double-Beef Burrito that I devoured in the car on the way home. I swore I would make better choices.

But looking back, I can't help but smile. Sure, I paid a hefty fee for my idiocy, but you can't put a price on a guy named Jake telling you, "You know, I really didn't want to like you when I found out Steph was engaged, but I can't help it. Be good to her."

I should have been resting. I should have stayed home. Instead, I jumped out of the nest and ignored everything I should have done. I was a honey badger.

Yay, me!

# 14

## CALL ME DOUCHEMAEL

I was not always the most considerate boyfriend. I blame my first girlfriend. Completely.

When I was sixteen, I met a girl at a party. (The party, coincidentally, was thrown by my friend Richard, the man who introduced me to Stephanie.) This girl was from the East Coast. She had traveled to St. Louis with her mom, who was on a business trip.

I had never had a ton of luck with women, so when this girl dared to talk to me, I thought it was only because she had no idea that I was the school geek with bad grades. I was the worst of the worst, but I happened to be friends with these cool new people she was meeting. We hung that night, and I left the party crestfallen. I knew I'd never see her again.

The next night, I went up to our local parish gym to play volleyball. Sunday night volleyball offered a nice opportunity for me to develop a shred of social skill. But that night, my heart wasn't in it; I couldn't get her out of my mind. I even rebuffed the invitation to Pantera's Pizza after the game. I headed home to hit fetal on my bed.

"Some girl called for you," my dad said when I walked through the door that night. "She left her number."

*A girl?*

"I think she's from out of town," he continued. "I didn't recognize the area code."

*Area code?*

I picked up the note my dad had scribbled. *Area code 201.* I called.

"Hello?" answered the sexiest phone voice I'd ever heard. It was her mother. Smoky, sultry pipes. I asked to speak to her daughter. (Historical note: this may have been the first time I hummed the *Jeopardy!* theme in my head.)

"Hello?"

"Hi. It's Dan."

She and I talked for half an hour that night.

Over the next nine months, my Sprint calling card bill averaged well over $250 a month, but I didn't care. I was in love like only a sixteen-year-old can be in love. "How can you be in love at sixteen?" skeptics may ask. Young as I was, it was the second most intense romantic love I've ever felt. It was raw, real, and unblemished by pain—because I was so young. Was it forever

## 14: CALL ME DOUCHEMAEL

love? No. But it was my first experience of really putting someone before myself.

I saw her two more times, each time for three days. I even flew her in for my junior prom. Her mom talked to my mom, and it was agreed that it was okay for her to stay at our house. She would sleep in the guest bedroom in our basement. I would sleep upstairs.

"She's an interesting woman," my mother said after hanging up. "She threatened your genitals if you two had sex."

My genitals would stay intact.

For our nine-month anniversary, I visited her on the East Coast on my way to Europe for a trip to see the Virgin Mary. (I'm not making this up.) We went to a very famous jewelry store where I bought her the least expensive token of my love that I could find. I was in love, but I was also on a budget.

Two days later, she broke up with me.

Devastated does not even begin to describe the brokenness of my heart. I was annihilated in a way I had never, ever known. I had laid myself bare before her altar, and she had sacrificed me on top of it with calculated scorn. From that day on, I swore I would never be hurt by a woman again. Ever.

Whenever I dated someone and I felt like it was going south, I'd immediately start to pull away. However, I didn't want to be a complete jerk about it, so the process would be gentle, almost glacial.

"I'm just gonna go out with my friends alone tonight. You don't mind, do you?"

"Of course not. See your friends," they would all say.

This was the beginning of the end. Making plans with my friends turned into calling less frequently—every other day, every third day, and so on. I'd start picking petty little fights. I'd shut down emotionally, slowly and methodically, which would, by design, cause the girl to hate me—and force her to do the dirty work of breaking up.

Or, if she wouldn't take the bait, I'd cut off all physical contact. A kiss goodbye would turn into a wave, and finally, once I couldn't take it anymore, I'd throw down the classic, "It's not you. It's me."

I was ghosting before ghosting was a thing.

And it really was me. I never started dating anyone with the intention of hurting that person. But I had built my walls so high and made them so impenetrable that no one ever had the chance to break through.

My grand designs never worked very well, though. As I started to pull away, the girl would hang on a little tighter. As I pulled harder, she would dig deeper. As I walked, she would follow, irritated. As I ran, she would throw a rock at the back of my head. "Where are you going? What just happened? Stop!"

But I was out of earshot. I could not, would not, hear. I was a jerk. And a coward.

I am grateful for the few women who agreed to give me a shot, and I regret hurting any of them. But I believe that your life is your life to live and no one else's. If you do for others just to make others happy, you will grow to resent them. And once you resent someone, it's almost impossible to reverse it.

I loved being my mom's baby again, and I loved that I was okay with letting her be my mom again. But once my doctor told me to enjoy week three, it was time to grow up. Or, in my case, leave my parents' house.

A year and a half prior, I left the *Steve and DC* radio show to pursue a career in film and video, and I was now a junior producer at a local video production company. My illness had placed my projects in the hands of other producers, but the one thing I could still do was teach. I was the main instructor for the StepStone Institute, the philanthropic wing of the production company. It was my job to teach at-risk young adults how to produce videos. I loved those kids, and I missed them terribly. When I felt strong enough to go to work, I jumped at the chance.

"I think I'm going to go into work today."

Gently, I started to pull away.

"Do you think that's a good idea?" My mother held on tighter.

"Yes, I do." I said, waving. "I love you!"

—

"Can I get you something to eat?"

I still hadn't gained very much weight, and my mom was frantic.

"I'm going over to Stephanie's. But thanks."

Tiptoeing away.

"You haven't brought her around in a while."

A dagger shot, well timed.

"I'll see if she'll come over this weekend."

Parry.

—

"Can I rub your head for you?"

My mom was looking for any foothold she could find.

"I'm okay for a head rub for now. But thanks, mom."

*Why is she still treating me like a baby?* My irritation began percolating through my forced politeness.

―

"Danny, you've been out every night. I want to see you stay home." My mom dug in.

"Mom, I'm not even supposed to be here. Leave me alone."

A shot to her soul.

Her eyes welled up as she walked out. She was silent.

"Mom…I'm sorry."

Nothing.

I heard her walk downstairs to her bedroom and softly close the door. The woman who gave me life; the woman who held me under her heart for nine months; the woman who had dropped everything in her life to take care of me; the woman who would have taken the cancer from my body and assumed it in her own; the woman who loved me like no one else ever would; that woman lay down on her bed and cried, for no other reason than my own selfishness.

I had broken both of our hearts, and it was a very, very long time before I forgave myself.

―

"Mom?"

Day four of my second round of chemotherapy. The first round of chemo was horrific beyond description. This was worse. I was scared. I wanted my mom.

"Mom?"

My bedroom door opened. My mom thought I looked like I was dying. She was right.

"Would you rub my head?"

## 14: CALL ME DOUCHEMAEL

In the throes of my suffering, it became harder and harder to smile, and not just from the chapped lips. Chemo subjected my body to a series of transmogrifications that caught me completely off guard.

One morning after getting out of the shower, I dried my face with a towel. When I looked down, I saw some short, wispy blonde hairs. These were peppered with some curved, thick, black ones.

"What the…?"

I looked in the mirror and discovered, to my horror, that my eyelashes and eyebrows were gone. I never knew that the lash lines of my eyelids were red. Bright red. It reminded me of the movie *Powder*. "He *is* electrolysis."

For the first time, I saw myself not as a sexy bald guy, but as a cancer patient. I was angry and scared and disgusted with my appearance. I didn't leave the house for three days.

When I finally felt well enough to visit my kids at the StepStone Institute, I wore a baseball cap and sunglasses, explaining that the sunlight was adversely affecting my vision, which was not a total lie.

A few days later, while I was waiting at an unnamed drive-through for my McChicken sandwich, a group of school kids—probably eight years old—walked out of the restaurant, presumably on a field trip. One of the kids locked eyes with me.

"Hi, bald guy!" he shouted.

The other kids thought this greeting was just a riot.

"Hi, bald guy!" "Hi, bald guy!" "Hi, bald guy!" The chorus echoed down the line.

I rolled down my window.

"I've got cancer, you little bastards!" I yelled as loudly as I could.

The next thing I knew, there were twenty-three screaming children and four very ticked-off teachers.

"You ought to be ashamed of yourself, scaring these kids!"

"Did you hear what they said to me?"

"How old are you?"

"I'm twenty-nine!" I screamed. "How old are you?"

According to her gesture, she was one.

When I made it back to StepStone and told my own students what had happened, they advised me to take a nap and then find Jesus.

# 15

## THE ELEPHANT

"So how did you get it?"
Chris was the first of maybe five people who have ever asked how I got cancer.

"I'm not sure. I think I just got it. It's not like you get ball cancer from smoking."

"Does it run in your family?"

"My grandpa had esophageal cancer, but he had GERD, and he smoked."

"So can you pass it on?"

This was a question I was not expecting.

"What do you mean 'pass it on?'"

"Well, if it's ball cancer, is your sperm tainted?"

"Umm…"

"It would make sense that it's tainted."

"I…guess?" *Tainted,* I thought. *Who uses the word* tainted? *Why is the word* tainted *so awful and appropriate?*

"So if you and Steph are…you know…and you finish…you know…could you infect her with your cancer?"

"She doesn't have balls, Chris."

"That's not my point. Could you pass it on like an STD since it started in your bag?"

When I was diagnosed with cancer, I didn't want anyone to treat me differently. I didn't have to worry about this with Chris. I had cancer? He didn't care. One time, he called and asked me to go to lunch. I told him I couldn't because I had to get a CT Scan and some blood work.

"You know, Duffy, it's always something with you."

*Click*

I wish everyone faced with cancer had a Chris. A Chris makes things easier. A Chris is there to disarm every situation. A Chris makes you feel normal, which is amazing since cancer is the most abnormal of situations.

I was blessed to be surrounded by so many friends and family members. I used to take it for granted; I don't anymore. Ever. I know so many people who have faced cancer alone, either because they didn't have a support system in place or because they didn't want to be a burden to anyone. For a long time, I belonged to the latter category.

"May I go downstairs and grab you a banana?" my mother asked.

"That's okay, Mom. I'll get it."

Only, I didn't get it, on any level. I didn't understand that my mom wanted nothing more than to be there for me, and to feel that I wanted and needed her there. It wasn't about the banana. It was a beautiful purpose, an expression of love. In my selfishness, I didn't want to be perceived as a burden. In her love, she wanted nothing more than to care for me.

My reluctance to receive help, and bananas, generated a vicious cycle, one that I didn't even see until it cracked me in the face.

A friend would ask if there was anything he could do for me. My response was mixture of thanks and anger. I was grateful the friend asked, but I reasoned that if I weren't sick, he wouldn't be asking. "No, but thanks anyway," I'd tell him, turning down his offering of kindness. If he persisted, I'd begin to resent him for treating me as though I were sick (even though I was sick).

Eventually, he'd pick up on the message I was laying down ("I don't want your freaking help!"), and he'd stop asking. Then, when I really did need the friend, I'd feel so guilty for turning down his assistance in the first place. I wouldn't ask for his help because I felt I didn't deserve it. Eventually, self-pity or self-preservation (or maybe both) would sculpt "I don't deserve it" into "He wouldn't help me anyway." And I'd begin to resent him for not being there for me.

It was insulation by isolation. I stopped going out. I stopped making calls. I stopped sending e-mails. I stopped talking to my family beyond the most topical of pleasantries, which by that time had become utterly unpleasant. I sulked, skulked, and tossed aside any semblance of the person they loved. They felt like they didn't know me anymore, and they certainly had no idea how to help. I made sure of that.

And before I knew it, I got my wish. I was utterly alone. I was alone on an island that I created. No shelter, no games, no animals, no fun. I was exiled with only my thoughts to keep me company. And my thoughts fell far short of comforting.

In my desolation, I became the master of self-flagellation. I beat the shit out of myself and scarred my own heart. I was incapable, I thought, of accepting anyone's love or compassion. I dug a hole, crawled in, and refused to come out. For the first time since shortly after my diagnosis, I was terrified. But this time, I wasn't afraid of dying.

I was afraid of living.

And then, out of nowhere, a most unexpected thing produced a most unexpected result.

I was sitting at an unnamed fine dining establishment, eating my Egg McMuffin, when my phone rang. I didn't recognize the number; the area code was from out of town.

"Hello?"

"Hey, Dan."

It was a friend who traveled a lot for work and whom I rarely saw. It was good to hear his voice.

"Hey, man! How are you?"

"I'm good, I'm good. Do you have a second?"

"Sure, what's up?"

There was a long pause on the line.

"I have to apologize to you."

"For what?"

"For not coming by to see you. For not calling you."

"Dude, don't worry about it." Since I had stopped talking to everyone, I hadn't even noticed that he didn't call.

"No, I need to say this."

## 15: THE ELEPHANT

I could hear him getting emotional on the line.

"You okay?" I asked.

"Dan, I don't know how to handle seeing you sick."

Honest. Brutal. Painful. Fantastic. I put down my rapidly cooling breakfast sandwich.

"It's the ostrich mentality. If I don't see you, you aren't sick. But I talked to Richard and Chris the other day, and they said you're in really bad shape."

"Oh, I'm not as bad as they think," I lied.

"Call them. They think you're dying."

And then it was my turn to break down, right in the middle of the restaurant. I had messed up so many things. I had kicked everyone out of my life, and I was terrified that no one would ever forgive me. I had no clue where to begin.

After my three minute sobbing *mea culpa*, he asked, "How do you eat an elephant, Dan?"

*Sniff.* "Excuse me…what?"

"How do you eat an elephant?"

"I have no idea."

"One bite at a time."

I knew my elephant well. The bastard was huge. It would take a lot of eating and require some crow mixed in for texture. But now, at least, I knew what to do. I would make things right, and I would take it one mouthful at a time.

It's amazing what a different perspective can give you: energy, drive, determination. I was fed up with being alone. I was fed up with loathing myself. I was fed up with being an asshole to those I loved. I was fed up with being miserable. I was mad as hell, and I wasn't going to take it anymore. I was going to get happy. Dammit.

My family made me eat only an ear's worth of metaphorical elephant before all was forgiven. My friends, on the other hand, made me choke down a lot more than that. And it wasn't from the end with the ear.

# 16

# MY BUCKET OF SUCK

I have always subscribed to the notion that, during chemo, it's the little things that propel you from day to day, the moments that fuel you when you don't have the energy to continue. These can be as simple as a smile from a friend, your red-hot fiancé mooning you, or discovering $20 in a coat you haven't worn in six months.

However, I'm also a proponent of having something huge to look forward to, and for me, that something was Ireland.

The year 2002 saw a lot of "5" and "0" birthdays in my family. My dad turned sixty; my uncle Declan, fifty; my cousin Orla, thirty; my grandmother, eighty-five; her sister, eighty. And I was turning thirty. We had planned the trip in 2001, before I was diagnosed.

That year—particularly, that summer—was going to be a global excursion. Not only were we supposed to go to Ireland in late May, but my dad was taking Gavin and me to the World Cup in South Korea less than a week after we got back from Ireland.

Thanks to cancer, we had to sell the quarterfinal and semifinal tickets back to the Korean Ticket Ministry. Thanks to my oncologist, however, Ireland was still a possibility.

The first two rounds of chemotherapy had shrunk my tumor by eighty-five percent. Treatment could not have gone any better. With this ammunition, I cautiously, tenderly, approached Dr. Needles.

"I'd like for you to postpone my last treatment by one week. I'm going to be out of town. It's non-negotiable."

Tact is my middle name.

"Dan, I don't know."

"It's Ireland. My parents are throwing a celebration party for a lot of family members and partly for me. Even the Australia cousins are flying in."

He picked up my chart and read it again.

"Well, I really couldn't be more pleased with your progress."

He put down the chart and looked at me dead in the eye.

"Please. This is important to me. I'll start the final round the day after I get back. I promise."

"How long?"

"Just a week."

"Alright. With the way you've responded, you're good."

"I'm going to need it in writing for my mom."

Dr. Needles shook his head and laughed. He knew. And I knew. All I had to do was get through round three and hello, Emerald Isle!

## 16: MY BUCKET OF SUCK

—

"I've never smoked the stuff, but if you're up for it, I'll do it with you. I'll even buy it. Where do I find a good hash dealer these days?"

Butter is a friend of ours, and we're not sure why. He has an amazing job. He has more letters *after* his name than *in* his name. He is crazy smart. And he lets us call him Butter, but not because he's smooth. He would have me murdered if I were to divulge why we call him Butter. To his wife, Isabel, I apologize.

He paid me a visit one day as I was suffering through the worst of round three's side effects. They were the same symptoms at rounds one and two, but these were a combination of the two. On crack. The nausea was amplified and constant. Simply rolling over in bed was enough to have me starring in the new play *Joseph and His Amazing Technicolor Yawn*. The chemo ate away at the nerves in my extremities like the fuse on a Yosemite Sam stick of dynamite, so my fingers and toes tingled incessantly. One of my ears would ring every twenty minutes for about twenty seconds each time. At the drop of a hat, sweat would actually stream out of my pores.

The drugs stopped working. To take the edge off chemo nausea, you are prescribed low-dose anti-psychotics. It starts with Ativan. When Ativan stops working, you get Zofran. When Zofran hits worthless, you try Zyprexa. And when that reaches failure…

You get Marinol, medicinal marijuana. Marinol is the Queen Mother of anti-nausea drugs. When Dr. Needles prescribed it, I wasn't sure what to expect. I thought it might be one of those big, horse-pill prescription bottles, only instead of pills, it would be filled with joints. Perhaps the label would read, "Puff, puff, pass every two hours for fast, effective relief. No refills."

Instead, I opened the cap and was greeted by a collection of small brown pellets that looked less like wonder drugs and more like rabbit turds. They were small, round, brown versions of Advil Liquigels. They were odorless, tasteless, worthless. All of the hallucinogenic properties that make pot…well…pot…were removed. As Cheech 'n' Chong would say, "That shit wouldn't get a fly high." And like all the others, it crashed and burned faster than poop through a goose. Years later, my oncologist would tell me that the drug never lived up to the promise of its hype.

And there was the rub. The anti-nausea drugs stopped working, and I had a lot of chemo to go. It scared, depressed, and angered me all at once, and I had had enough. I reached the point that my friend Robert Schimmel (God rest him) told me he had experienced during his own battle with cancer: "You know you're not going to die, but you want to."

Yet even in my complete and total misery, I was so humbled that Butter, a guy who has never smoked the stuff and who has to take random drug tests at work, would throw caution to the wind to help me in any way he could.

"Thanks, Butter," I said, "but I'm going to have to pass on your offer."

"You sure? My treat."

I had my reasons for turning down a chance to dance with Mary Jane free of charge.

Years ago, during one of our better family trips to Bermuda, Gavin and I, along with some friends from New Jersey, were hanging by the pool after dark. A Rasta we had seen earlier in the day walked up to us and said "hello."

"Is that pot?" I asked.

"Pure Bermuda Gold, man. Wanna heet?"

## 16: MY BUCKET OF SUCK

I had not experimented a lot with pot, but I'd partaken a few times. The first time was on my seventeenth birthday. I invited some people over, and one of my friends, Scott, brought over a new guy I'd never met.

"Brian. Nice to meet you."

As we were talking, he produced a dugout from his pocket.

"Time to swing the bat."

"Swinging the bat" meant stuffing a small brass pipe into the opening of a wooden container inspired by the Grateful Dead.

"Want one?" asked my new friend.

It was the first of maybe ten times in my life when I smoked pot. Was I a wake-n-baker? Hardly. But I can't say I really hated it, either. So the thought of burning one on vacation seemed like a fine idea. What could go wrong?

"Sure, let's see what this island has to offer," I told the Rasta.

Four heets and twenty minutes later, while reclining on a chaise lounge, the sky began to spin. I mean, *the whole thing*. Stars were no longer stars; they were white circles of glow. You know Van Gogh's *Starry Night*? Picture it alive, moving at ludicrous speed. This was my new reality. After only a few heets.

I'm not sure how my brother got me off the chaise. He probably had to pry it out of my ass, which was balled up like a fist. I don't remember walking through the lower lobby. I don't remember the elevator to the fourth floor. I don't remember getting into bed. All of these memories were superseded by hyperventilation.

Never before had I feared for my life more than I did that night. My pulse was at least one-eighty for two hours, minimum. I couldn't slow my breathing. Even Gavin was terrified for me. He kept bringing cold washcloths to put on my head.

"God, if you let me live," I prayed, "I'll never touch the stuff again. I promise. Please just let me live."

And I meant it.

I don't know when I passed out, but when I woke up, I felt my body, my clothes, the bed, and anything else I could get my hands on. Was I dead? Was this heaven?

"Dude, the next time you do that, I'll kill you, myself."

Gavin was pissed. This was definitely hell.

"I won't."

Years had passed, but I was going to keep my promise.

"I appreciate it, Butter, but I can't for religious reasons."

"Oh, I'm sure Jesus got high from time to time."

"You're probably right," I said.

—

I worked hard to get my head out of my funk, and around friends and family at least, I was a bit more successful. What I couldn't get past was my tendency to look behind me. After I finished my second round of chemo, I was hopeful. *I'm half done!* I told myself. *Half done. Only half more to go!*

But when the side effects of round three kicked in, I did not look to the future. I started looking backwards. *I'm only a little over half done. Only half done. I don't think I can go on.*

Runners call this "hitting the wall."

I called it "my bucket of suck."

The effects of chemotherapy are cumulative. Every cancer patient knows this all too well. Round one is harder than anything you can imagine. Round two is even worse. Round three is a special kind of hell.

## 16: MY BUCKET OF SUCK

Nausea hit me harder. Fatigue hit me harder. Pain hit me harder. Hell, I looked balder. Harold Tango Foxtrot is that even possible? By the end of my fifteenth treatment, all I could do was cling to anything that was positive and tangible. I leaned heavily on Stephanie. I admired her strength; I was stronger because of it. I was blessed to have someone who didn't look at me like I was about to die, even if she felt it.

My mom tried not to think of my mortality, but she couldn't help it. Even for a sick person, I looked sick. I knew it crushed her to see me in this state, so I forced myself to get out occasionally—even if "getting out" simply meant stepping outside for some air—just to show her that I wasn't dead yet.

It's hard to watch someone you love hurting so badly. I can't imagine watching someone I love on the brink of death. I will always sympathize, but I hope to never empathize.

Years later, she told me that once, when I was at my sickest, she went up to my room to straighten it up. She sat on the edge of my bed and picked up the blanket I used to combat night shivers. She brought it up to her nose. It smelled like me.

She then fell to the floor and screamed for five solid minutes. My dad came racing up the stairs to see if she had hurt herself, but her pain came from somewhere far deeper than bone and muscle. She had her emotional breakdown, and she waited for me to be out of the house before she had it.

To this day, I thank God that she embraced it, and I thank God that I didn't see it.

For the first time since my initial diagnosis, my mother questioned whether I was going to live or die. That's the double-edged sword of chemotherapy. It brings you to the brink of extinction without actually taking your life. Even then, it's a very, very fine line. Depending on the severity or aggressiveness of the cancer, an oncologist has to throw everything he or she can at the cancer to kill it and somehow manage not to kill you in the process.

Someday, this will change. There are new treatments on the horizon, things we can't even imagine. I was on a plane and met an amazing man named Xiaobin (pronounced SHOW-bin). Xiaobin was a graduate student at Yale and was working on targeted treatment of cancer cells based on a person's DNA. This was in 2013. God only knows how far they've come since then.

When I received treatment, there was no such medical breakthrough. My chemo was akin to a blitzkrieg: it destroyed everything in sight, everything on both my Western and Eastern Fronts. It was a carpet-bombing of Dresden proportions. All I could do was hang on for dear life. It wasn't, "This is going to be unpleasant." It was, "Oh. My. God."

I'll never forget what Dr. Larry Einhorn, the man who pioneered my therapy, said to Lance Armstrong before treating him. Lance told Dr. Einhorn, "Throw everything at me. Kill me if you can." Dr. Einhorn responded that they would do everything to cure him: "And I can kill you."

This was my existence. The light at the end of my tunnel was another freight train. And another. And another. I no longer thought about going to Ireland in two weeks. I didn't know if I would make it. I didn't care.

I just wanted everything to go away.

Even me.

# 17

## GOING HOME

"I didn't think I'd see this."

I held Stephanie's hand and rested my bald head against her flowing red tresses. Outside the airplane window, four thousand feet below us, forty shades of green reflected the sunlight in all its glory. I was home.

Dr. Needles had examined me with a fine-toothed comb. My white blood cells were back and better than ever. My appetite returned, as four extra pounds proved. My energy hadn't been this electric since I felt the pain for the first time. And I produced enough natural gas to power Rhode Island. Passengers complained. There was nothing I could do.

I had survived round three. The first morning that I didn't feel like regurgitating my shoes was a revelation. If I could survive round three, I could survive anything. Sure, round four would be worse physically, but it would be the last round, and the last round is when you hold nothing back. You leave it all on the track. Or the field. Or the mat. Or your bathroom floor.

I also knew that I would not have to endure a round five. According to my last CT scan, there was no noticeable trace of my tumor. The chemo had worked, and while I cursed it for being the bastard it is, I gave it a high five for a job well done.

"It's so beautiful," Stephanie agreed.

She had been to Ireland with her friend, Kelly, as a college graduation present. They took a bus tour, and their youth brought the average age of the bus tourists down to seventy-four. They were the last ones to go to bed each night and the last ones to climb aboard before the bus left each morning. Good—*hiccup*—times.

I was giddy for so many reasons. Our hotel was a stone's throw from St. Stephen's Green, a park in the heart of Dublin City where my mom used to take me to feed the ducks as a little boy. I'm nostalgic like that.

And the room was fantastic, massive for Ireland standards. The bed was huge, the bathroom was marble, and our view faced the city. I opened the windows as soon as we walked in and inhaled the air, a lovely mixture of bus exhaust, burning peat, the Guinness brewery, and the color green.

Yes, green is a scent in Ireland.

My cousin Emer had already left a message at the hotel for us. She and her fiancé, Alan, whom we were meeting for the

## 17: GOING HOME

first time that night, would see us in the hotel lobby at six. We'd catch up over a glass of wine before walking to the Imperial, a Chinese restaurant that has been around, in one form or another, for over fifty years. It was at the end of Wicklow Street, just around the corner from Trinity College. The Imperial has the best beef curry I've ever had, and I'd been salivating at the thought of having it for weeks. By the time we got to Chicago, our lone stopover between St. Louis and Dublin, I could contain myself no longer.

"Only nineteen hours 'til curry!" I squealed to Stephanie on the flight across the ocean.

"You are a freak," she smiled.

Alan had already ordered a bottle of wine for the table by the time Steph and I made our way to the lobby bar. He was a handsome devil with a wit that reminded me of my brother: slightly biting, brilliantly simple. They both see things a tick on the askew side, something I envy and admire.

Emer was the first to greet us. *The first relative to see me bald*, I thought with a shudder.

"Look at you, gorgeous!" she said.

Emer: 1. Self-consciousness: nil.

Even though we had seen each other only once every three or four years since I moved from Ireland, Emer and I had a close relationship. When I finally met Alan, I was thrilled such an amazing guy had swept her off her feet.

And I was so touched with how they took to the woman who had swept me off of my feet. Steph had now met the first two members of my extended family.

"I love them," she whispered in my ear, stealing a moment during the conversation.

My brother Gavin joined us in the lobby. His wife, Alison, who was very pregnant at the time, had stayed in St. Louis. Gavin would be the third wheel on our tricycle of awesome.

The five of us spent the better part of an hour making each other laugh. No one said a single word about my medical situation. For the first time in a long time, I didn't think about needles (spikey or Doctor) or chemo or pain or puking. In fact, puking was the furthest thing from my mind. I was starving for curry. I looked at my watch.

"Let's do this."

---

*Snap!*

A member of the Chinese triad called the waiter to his table with the flick of two fingers. The server ran over, face down to avoid eye contact, and removed the soiled plates before another server immediately brought a fresh plate to the table.

For ninety minutes, we took turns sneaking glances at this mountain of a man. He had thinning black hair, shaded eyeglasses, a black suit, a large pinky ring, and the demeanor of Tony Soprano. He was terrifying.

He ate as though eating was the sole purpose of his existence. I've never seen anyone order so much food, and he did it all without speaking a word. The pitch of his snaps informed the staff of his every need.

Apparently, the Imperial was popular with *Chinese* Chinese food lovers, too.

We kept to ourselves, laughing, looking, drinking, and looking some more. I ordered my beef curry mild with fried rice and a

## 17: GOING HOME

side of fries, or chips as they call them. So did Gavin. Beef curry. Fried rice. Chips. Stephanie ordered the same. She wanted to see what all the fuss was about.

Twenty minutes later, the food arrived. Stephanie spooned rice onto her plate, plucked approximately five pieces of beef and onion, and gently napped it on top of the rice.

With uncouth flourish, Gavin and I dumped our rice on our plates and dumped the curry over the rice. I then almost stabbed our server in the hand when she tried to take away the sauce remnants on my silver curry platter.

"Dipping chips," I explained. She apologized in five different languages.

And then I began eating, and I never came up for air. At one point, I sneezed, and two grains of rice flew out of my nose. I ordered a second plate of chips. They were the best chips I'd ever had.

*Snap!*

The waiter raced back over to Paulie Walnuts, but this time, he pointed his bratwurst-sized finger to our table.

Oh shit; we'd insulted him…somehow. Maybe we weren't supposed to dip the chips? Maybe we were being too loud? Maybe we were going to be murdered?

A minute later, a penitent server delivered a plate of chips and a bowl of curry sauce to his table.

*Dip. Slurp. Chew.*

Well played, Big Pussy.

Ireland should have a sign that says, "Thank you for smoking." In the nineties, people used to light up on the tarmac while waiting to disembark from the plane. Most indoor spaces throughout the country felt like a Rush concert. The moment you walked through the door, you were smacked across the lungs with tobacco smoke.

So I was baffled when I opened the door to the *Café en Seine*, our next port of call after the Imperial, and smelled…*nothing*.

"Where's the smoke?"

"Ireland is smoke-free in most indoor places now," Alan said.

"Wow! When did that happen?" I asked.

"Months ago."

Stephanie was ecstatic. I didn't mind it either. We each had two drinks to celebrate.

---

We eventually found ourselves in the Temple Bar area of Dublin. Temple Bar boasts about two hundred restaurants and pubs—and just as many ways to get in trouble. I don't remember the bar we went to, but I do remember a shot. And a beer. And another shot.

---

"We've gotten a room. Come down for a nightcap."

Emer and Alan were far too blotto to drive, so they did what any self-respecting couple would do: they booked a room in our hotel and bought a bottle of wine in the lobby bar. They then invited us to their room to help them consume said bottle of wine. I couldn't have piloted a Big Wheel at that point, and I needed

# 17: GOING HOME

more liquor like Richard Simmons needs shorter shorts. But, hey, we were on vacation. I was playing hooky from chemo—with my doctor's permission. If I was going to vomit, it was going to be due to the imbecilic choices I made, not the choices made for me. *Think you're bad, Cisplatin? Meet my friend Jim Beam. (Mic drop.)*

—

3:45 a.m. Emer and Alan were asleep in one bed. Stephanie and I were in the other. She was sleeping, sprawled across the bed diagonally. I was not…too busy trying to get comfortable on the mattress toast point that was left for me. Not happy.

—

5:53 a.m. I heard Emer and Alan shuffling out the door. I passed out again.

—

9:40 a.m. "Shit!"
I fell off the edge of the bed and leapt to my feet.
"Steph! Wake up! We're late!"
Stephanie cracked opened her eyes.
"What…oh, no!"
She jumped out of bed. We shot out of Emer and Alan's room like a canon blast and raced back to our own, where five messages awaited us.

Before the trip, my mother had asked Steph and me if we wanted to do anything special. We thought it would be fun to explore the country a bit. My folks hired a driver who would collect Steph, Gavin, and me and ferry us to the west, near Galway. The driver was scheduled to pick us up at 9:00 a.m. That morning. It was now 9:46.

I knew my parents would be frantic. I clicked the button next to the blinking light on the hotel phone and held my breath.

"Hi, Danny. It's your mother," the first message began. "It's a few minutes before nine. Just letting you know we're here. See you soon. Love you!"

The breakdown occurred over the next four.

"Danny! Danny! I'm so worried!" wailed the final message. "I don't know if you're dead! I don't know if you're in jail! You're not in your room! Stephanie might be wandering the streets by herself! Oh, Jesus, I'm going to call the morgue!"

Very rarely in my adult life have I been truly scolded by my parents. At 9:57 a.m., in the lobby of the Conrad Hotel, I got my ass chewed like the main prop in a Skoal commercial.

After the tongue-lashing, they composed themselves.

"Can we get a picture before you go?" asked my mother.

Leaving the hustle and bustle of the city and driving through the serenity of the countryside, I can't say I felt good on any level. I was hung over, I had disappointed my parents, I had been (deservedly) lectured in front of Stephanie, and I had my picture taken, which may have been the worst of all.

From age thirteen to fifteen, I made my solitary ambition in life to avoid getting my picture taken. I was half human, half Transformer, equipped with the kind of braces that fit all the way around your teeth. I hated them with my soul. To make sure I'd never have to see them again once they came off, I refused to show my teeth in any of the few pictures that people did manage

# 17: GOING HOME

to take. You will not find a single picture of me during that time with my teeth showing. Not one.

I felt the same way about being bald. It wasn't something I wanted to remember. It was the ostrich mentality in past tense. If there is no evidence, did it really happen?

The picture my mom took that morning was the second and final picture snapped of me during treatment. And it was the only picture of me in Ireland.

As bad as things got during my four months of hell there were some good times as well. Great times. Beautiful memories. With friends. With family. And I have only two pictures to show for it. This scares me because without tangible, visible reminders of the past, memories fade. For that incredible trip to Ireland, I have almost nothing to hold on to.

I couldn't get out of the way of my own self-consciousness. It's one of the very few regrets that I will carry with me forever.

# 18

## THE CELEBRATION OF LIFE

We drove through the back roads in the west of Ireland. The landscape was a maze of short stone walls, overwooled sheep, and shades of green that redefined the color spectrum. As my hangover had recently abated, I couldn't help but smile at all that had transpired in the past twelve hours.

The hotel my mother had booked for us was not a hotel at all. It was a large, eight-bedroom manor house named St. Claren's that was once the family home of the legendary director John Huston.

The rooms didn't even have numbers; they had names. Each one was massive, with a bed so luxurious that a Saudi Arabian sheikh, who visited the house a few months before we did, woke up after his first night and offered $25,000 for the bed—as is—to be brought back to his kingdom.

In typical Irish fashion, the ladies who run St. Claren's politely refused; they did, however, write out an entire list detailing how to create the bed from scratch, from mattress to pillows to feather beds to sheets. They even threw in where to buy the supplies at a discount. Probably saved the guy well over twenty grand.

Dinner was at seven, but Stephanie and I left our room an hour early to explore the house a bit. As we came down the stairs, one of the ladies asked if we would like a glass of wine before dinner.

"That would be lovely," we said in unison.

She walked us into a drawing room and asked us to take a seat on a couch in front of the fireplace. Before our butts hit the cushions, she lit a match and started a fire. The smell of the burning peat bricks was a thing of glory.

For over an hour, we sat on the couch, sipping our wine, smelling the fire, feeling the warmth, listening to the birds outside the open window, melting into the comfort of each other. All five senses were working in rare and perfect harmony. I didn't want it to end.

"How long have you been down here?" asked Gavin as he walked into the room, thirty seconds before dinner.

"Not long enough," I said. "What have you been doing?"

"The same thing I did the entire ride here."

"Sleeping," Stephanie and I said together.

"Did you feel that bed? That's a holy shit bed," said Gavin. I told him the sheikh story.

"Totally getting that bed when I get back," he said.

The ladies came in and brought us to the dining room. *Time to Say Goodbye* by Andrea Bocelli and Sarah Brightman filled the air as the first course came out, a savory morsel wrapped in puff pastry.

"I'm starving," I said, picking it up with my hand and shoving it into my mouth. In retrospect, I really should have asked what was *in* the puff pastry.

Immediately, my eyes misted. My nervous system sent panic signals down to my toenails. My jaws, somehow, locked themselves shut. Writhing in agony, my teeth clenched despite my greatest efforts to separate them, I used my tongue to force the rest of the sheep spleen down my throat. My stomach, assuming my esophagus had launched an assault, rejected the pastry and sent it spewing forth.

In one grand eruption, sheep spleen exploded from every facial orifice I had (including, I am certain, my eyes) and onto the table in front of me. Stephanie thought I was dying. Gavin was dying from laughing. And every single patron at every other table looked at me like I was a member of the Chinese triad.

A minute later, I retrieved my dignity from the floor as my face returned to an acceptable level of crimson.

"So, would you or would you not recommend them?" Gavin asked.

"You are an asshole."

—

As we walked back to our room from what was otherwise an exceptional meal, I silently said a prayer of thanks to God. That He would spare me to enjoy an evening like this was a gift, and

I told Him that I would try to be a more grateful person from that point on.

When we got back to our room, we found our bed turned down, the lights muted, and the speaker system softly cooing Irish music.

I was grateful indeed. It would be hard to leave this place. If I had been smart, I would have taken lots of pictures. But sometimes, I am not smart.

Sometimes, I am a dumbass.

—

When we pulled up to the Green Isle Hotel that Saturday evening, a torrent of memories came flooding back to me. My parents used to have dinner parties there whenever we would come back from the States for a visit. The reunions. The food. The hotel. Even at twenty-nine, I was a sentimental old fool.

My mom's dad, Paddy, had died when she was pregnant with me. My mom's mom, my Nannie, remarried in 1981. Her second husband, Eddie, was the closest thing to a maternal grandfather I ever had.

Nannie and Eddie's wedding reception was at the Green Isle Hotel. Nannie was exceptionally stylish in a light yellow dress and a matching yellow hat that wrapped around her head. I remember my dad dancing with her to *Annie's Song* by John Denver, which our family henceforth called "Nannie's Song."

I also remember that we would always bring gifts for our relatives when we made a trip back to the Motherland. One of the staples was a box of King Edward cigars for Eddie. Then, when my parents and I would bring Nannie and Eddie to the Green

## 18: THE CELEBRATION OF LIFE

Isle for dinner, he would have half the box stuffed into his jacket, ready to hand out to every male worker at the hotel.

The *maître d'* at the Green Isle was a man named Bobby. Bobby made sure that we were all treated like royalty. He had a soft spot in his heart for Eddie, and when Eddie would shove a cigar into his hand, Bobby was genuinely grateful, even though, as far as we knew, Bobby never smoked a day in his life. Even if Bobby's entire gene pool had been killed off by lung cancer, he still told Eddie, "Ah, Jaysus! I'll enjoy that one later!" Bobby always made a special fuss of Eddie.

And boy was a fuss made when we went home in 1993 to throw Eddie a ninetieth birthday celebration at the Green Isle. Eddie was so drunk on Bobby's steady stream of brandy and white sparkling lemonades that my parents made me follow him every time he went to the toilet, just to make sure he didn't fall in.

These were also the days before Flomax. Peeing took a while for a ninety-year-old.

Invariably, whenever it was time for Eddie to leave, he'd have one cigar left of the twenty he packed in his suit coat specifically to give away. It was a tradition to complain that the men took all his cigars.

"Mother of Christ, Danny, do you believe those robbers?"

"Thieves, Eddie. Nothing but thieves."

—

My dad's mom, Tess, my Nana, was the queen mother of matriarchs. She was the definitive head of the Duffy clan, a loving woman, but not the cuddliest babe on the block. Strong and fiercely

Catholic, she was not above verbal crucifixion. As Gavin put it, "She carries the hammer and nails around in her purse."

On the night of the *Celebration of Life* party, Nana sat next to her sister, Eileen, both of whom were welcoming milestone birthdays, eighty-five and eighty, respectively. While only five years apart in age, the two were generations apart in attitude. Eileen, the younger sister, had moved to New York years before and subsequently found herself a single mother of more children than I can remember.

Instead of sulking in self-pity, Eileen worked more jobs at one time than I've had in my entire life. She showered her children with love, and they adored her. By the time she retired to Florida with her husband Dick (also a testicular cancer ass-kicker), four of her children followed suit just to remain close to her.

Eileen still colored her hair, dressed like a movie star, and danced more than anyone else that night. She was a spectacular woman, and she fell in love with Stephanie instantly.

Nana also liked Stephanie. In fact, at the moment, she probably liked her more than she liked me.

"You didn't come to visit me," she said. Indicted, right in the middle of dinner.

"I'm sorry, Nana. We were out of town."

"You got back on Thursday. You could have come to visit me."

"I know, Nana."

"Well, if you know, then why didn't you visit me?" She pursed her lips and shook her head condemningly for a good thirty seconds.

I didn't avert my gaze. I held my ground.

She didn't avert her gaze. She held her ground.

Emer, who was sitting next to Stephanie, made a fist with her face to keep from laughing.

"Welcome to the family," she whispered to my fiancé.

Nana and I continued our stare down. No one at the table said a word. Between the occasional bells ringing in my ears, I heard the faint showdown whistle from *The Good, The Bad, and the Ugly*. *I've seen hell the past few months*, I thought. *My will is like a piece of iron. You are not winning tonight, Nana.*

"How was the west, Daniel?"

God love you, Eileen. Nana was waiting to flog me at the slightest twitch, and her own sister gave me an out.

"It was wonderful, Eileen. The food was lovely, the bed was unlike anything I've ever slept in, and Steph and I had some of the best *alone* time we've ever had. It was epic."

Emer spit water out of her mouth.

Stephanie kicked me in the shin.

"Sacred heart of the Divine Redeemer!" screamed Nana.

Eileen gave me a sly smile. God, I loved that woman.

—

I have to hand it to my father. He pulled out every stop for our *Celebration of Life* gathering in Ireland. He looked up all of the old relations from Ireland, England, America, and even Australia. And they all came.

Eileen brought her husband, Dick, from Melbourne, Florida. My mom's sister, Nora, came from Portsmouth, England. Of course, all of my cousins and aunts and uncles from Dublin were there. And about twenty people made the trek all the way from Australia.

But the highlight for my dad was calling up all of the "5" and "0" birthdays. There were eight of us, including my uncle Declan, my cousin Orla, my Nana, my great aunt Eileen, and my father himself. I was the last one called up. My father gave a short but eloquent speech about his vision for our trip. He said when he first planned it, he never imagined the name *Celebration of Life* would be so appropriate.

Through his words, I finally saw what I had suspected: my cancer gutted him. My father is a very loving man, but he doesn't always verbalize his sentiments. That night, maybe for the first time, he did.

I was so moved, but so uncomfortable at the same time. Everyone at the gathering now knew how close I came to death. If my cancer had not been diagnosed when it was, I would have died before I knew what hit me.

Plus, I wasn't exactly looking my best. My eyebrows and eyelashes had fallen out in the shower (again) that evening while I was getting ready, and even though I felt great, I still looked sick. Yes, I loved being surrounded by so much love, but I worried about being pitied.

As it turned out, no one pitied me. Rather, they rallied me. They knew I would be starting more chemotherapy in three days and that it would be my last round.

"We're praying for you," Aunt Patricia said.

"Kick its fucking arse," Aiden from Australia ordered.

Every ten minutes, I'd get a shot of courage and support. I walked out of the Green Isle on fire. I was ready. I could take on hell one last time.

But hell could wait. We still had one last day in Ireland.

## 18: THE CELEBRATION OF LIFE

"We have to get out of Ireland. Now," my dad informed us over the phone. "Come to our room."

It was the morning after the *Celebration of Life*, and I had planned a little breakfast in bed for Steph and I. My best laid plans of mice, men, and Eggs Benedict would just have to wait. Stephanie and I ran up the hall to meet my parents. We had no idea what was going on.

"Aer Lingus is on strike."

"But we're flying British Airways to London," said Gavin who had arrived a minute before us.

"But the flight is run by Aer Lingus," replied my dad.

"Which means what?" I asked.

"Which means if we can't get to London somehow by tomorrow morning, we can't get home, and you can't start chemotherapy on Tuesday."

*Oh, shit.*

"If you aren't packed, go pack. Now."

Stephanie and I raced back to our room and began throwing everything into our suitcases, jumping on them like trampolines to get them closed. As soon as we finished, the phone rang again.

"Here's the plan," my dad directed. "In two hours, we're getting a lift to the ferry terminal. We'll get on the ferry, and then it's two and a half hours to Holyhead."

"Where's Holyhead?"

"Wales. A driver will pick us up there and drive us down to Heathrow."

"How far is that?"

"About four and a half hours."

"Jesus."

"Then we'll get a motel and grab a few hours of sleep before we fly home from Heathrow in the morning."

"Is this the only way?" I asked. The whole ordeal sounded awful.

"Yes."

And I thought jetlag was going to be the worst of my traveling issues.

---

A stag party. Awesome.

A contingent of British lads realized that Ireland does everything better and, that being the case, decided to give their engaged mate one last hurrah on the Emerald Isle. This was the last leg of their trip.

And they were all drunk. And they were on our ferry.

---

Have you ever seen *Deadliest Catch* on Discovery Channel? You know when the crew of The Northwestern has to battle twenty-foot swells while trying to pull a pot full of crab onto the deck, as Mother Nature smacks them with salt and spray and the occasional ball-shrinking cold rogue wave, causing the grizzled old deck boss to inadvertently impale his hand through a railing cleat, prompting the greenhorn to puke all over the cameraman in the corner, leading to Captain Sig to light up yet another cigarette while tapping his feet steering the boat and lamenting about life on the Bering Sea?

## 18: THE CELEBRATION OF LIFE

I knew their pain. And after the ferry ride, so did the British lads, who were now vomiting in glorious display.

—

I didn't know that when you bring luggage on a ferry, you have to go through the same process as you do at the airport. You check your bags at departure, you complete your journey, and then you retrieve your luggage from a conveyor belt.

I also didn't know that one of the British lads must have checked himself on a dare. But there he was, coming down the conveyor belt with the rest of the luggage.

And he was naked. And his bare ass was spitting distance from my suitcase.

I wish I were making this up.

—

Gavin was ashen. He, Stephanie and I were wedged into the very last row of seats of a minivan heading from Wales to London. Our driver was a twenty-something *GQ* model. Gavin glanced at the speedometer and then smacked me on my knee. My gaze shifted from *Notting Hill*, which was playing on the DVD screen above us, to my petrified brother.

"Do you know how fast we're going?" he asked.

"Uh-uh."

"A buck thirty-five."

"Kilometers?"

Gavin slowly shook his head from side to side.

It was supposed to take four and a half hours from Holyhead to Heathrow. Mario Andretti got us there in a tick under three.

—

My father traded frequent flyer miles to get us back to the states in first class. It was an amazing gesture and cap to what turned out to be one of the best vacations of my life—and the one for which I was most grateful.

I was also grateful that it was the summer time, so there was no worry about getting grounded on the tarmac in a snowstorm for nine hours again. Once in a lifetime is once too many for an experience like that.

Stephanie and I had switched seats so she could sit by the window. Twenty minutes before departure, the flight attendant walked up to us and offered us a beverage.

"May I get you something, miss?"

"I would love a glass of champagne," Stephanie said.

The flight attendant looked at her list of passengers before addressing me.

"And can I get something for you, Mr. Wrigley?"

From the row in front of us, my father exploded in laughter.

"Get used to that, Mr. Wrigley."

# 19

## BARTENDER! ONE MORE ROUND!

Few things in my life have made me feel ballsier than going to my last rounds of chemotherapy. True, the worst of the physical suffering was still ahead of me; this was certain. But I couldn't wipe the perma-grin off my face. The emotional suffering—the hardest part—was over.

Throughout treatment, as much as the chemo wreaked havoc on my body, it did an even bigger number on my psyche. The emotional agony compounded the physical. Not having to deal with the former during the final round was a huge relief.

Life always moves forward, whether you like it or not, so if you're looking backwards, you're going to hit something—whether it be a block, a wall, or an open manhole. During the worse part of my chemo, round three, I looked backwards, and I fell through my fair share of open manholes because of it.

But now I was in the home stretch, and there was no stopping my momentum. Day one was a snap. I sat in the chair for four hours and took my medicine. I even held out from peeing for the second time. I took it as a win.

Day two was even easier. I slept the entire time. I had purposely stayed up late the night before so that I'd be a zombie by the time I got to the chair. Save for a quick pee halfway through, I had an amazing nap.

Day three was a cakewalk. A couple of friends showed up, and before I knew it, I was halfway done. I even chatted with the nurses, many of whom only knew me as "the sourpuss in the corner who never talked." They turned out to be really, really nice people.

Even a few members of the Old Guard, most of whom I had seen since the start of my treatment, gave me a thumbs up as I walked out. They could tell my sentence was almost finished, and they were genuinely happy for me. *I should have talked to them more*, I thought. *Maybe tomorrow.*

And then tomorrow came. *Day four.*

*Oh, my God.*

I was on mile nineteen of a twenty-mile marathon, and I hit the wall, a lead-lined, cinderblock wall. And I was wearing a turbo-model jetpack when I hit it. And it was turned on.

I thought I had an idea of how bad the last rounds of chemo would be, but I was blindsided by just how horrendous it was. The chemo drugs started playing with my head. I'm not sure how

## 19: BARTENDER! ONE MORE ROUND!

I avoided this side effect during the earlier rounds, but in this last bout, it was heets of "Pure Bermuda Gold" all over again, and no prayer was getting me out of it.

The nausea was only the tip of the iceberg. My toes and fingers tingled constantly, and not even the good kind of tingle you get after…you know…an amazing session of…well…you know. This tingle was a pins-and-needles tingle. I felt like my nerves were being eaten alive.

I stopped pooping again. So there's that. I also had one hot flash per hour, on average. I'm a sweater by nature. During each episode, my forehead literally poured perspiration, and my pants filled with body broth (at least, it felt that way). I showered three times a day to combat the odor. I had to stop using antiperspirant because blocking sweat in one area just made it go to another area. [See: *swamp ass.*]

I thought I was beyond embarrassment. I had endured every indignity you could possibly imagine. I had been poked, prodded, ball-trasounded. Twice. But the wreck of humanity that stared back at me in the mirror was too much. I looked like death regurgitated. When I showed up for my second-to-last day of chemo, I ducked my head in to tell the nurses I had arrived, found my chair, and promptly pulled the curtain around me. I didn't want anyone to see my hideousness.

But neither cancer nor the chemo bent on its destruction cared about my appearance. In fact, they had one last adventure in store.

We got back from Ireland on a Monday, which meant that my last five treatments were from Tuesday through Saturday. And because the infusion center wasn't open on the weekend, the fifth treatment would take place in a hospital, which meant that I would have to be admitted for the day.

I shared a semi-private room with a fifty-year-old gout victim. At the time, I didn't know what gout was. By the end of the day, I knew I could have lived my entire life perfectly content not to know what gout was.

Furthermore, the cavalcade of visitors who came by to hang with my gouty roommate had bordered on ridiculous. People brought him flowers. Young children pulled on his gouty feet in wonder. And there was a magic show. *A magic show.*

*And what the hell is that clown doing here? Wait...I think he's got a gun!*

My chemo-head was worse than I thought.

My final treatment also marked the first time Stephanie was able to go to an appointment with me. As a final-year pharmacy student, she spent much of her time completing rotations and working at a local pharmacy. She had never been able to come to one of my treatments, which meant she had never been able to see me in this condition. In some ways, I was relieved that she hadn't. However, on this last day, I welcomed her visit. It's one thing to sit in a recliner for a few hours and take a nap. It's quite another to spend a few hours in a hospital bed watching *Bring Me Back My Baby* on the Lifetime Channel next to someone dying of gout.

*I bet she kidnapped her own baby. And how she's all, "Someone stole my baby!" And she's going to get insurance money and fall in love with the investigator until he busts her for being a baby murderer. Baby murderer!*

Delirium dug in. I turned my vitriol to the gout victim.

*And what the hell is gout anyway? And what makes Gouty McGoutenstein so special? Look at the fuss they're making of him! Well fuck him, and fuck his gout! Gout! Who gets flowers for gout? I didn't know it was red roses for love, yellow roses for friendship, and white roses for...fucking...gout! I didn't even know gout existed anymore! How much of a dick do you have to be to get stricken with a previously eradicated disease? Fucker!*

As was so often the case, Stephanie was the one who talked me off the ledge. Seeing her walk through the door was akin to an instantaneous slap back to reality.

"Hi baby" I said, not daring to alert her to my potentially gouticidal thoughts.

She came over to the bed, kissed me, and got in next to me. Having her there was enough to calm my fears, and my psychosis for that matter. She held my hand and ate my broccoli florets. We laughed, we dreamed, and we thanked God that this was it for chemotherapy.

But the visit was fleeting. Her brother Pat and his wife Tiffiny had just had their first child, Kira, while we were in Ireland. Steph was going to see her niece for the first time, and she was thrilled. When it was time for her to leave, she felt guilty about having to go, but I assured her that she had made the day extraordinary and that we would celebrate when I felt better.

She walked out the door. I felt completely and utterly alone. Goutboy had passed out. His visitors were gone. I stared blankly at the television, cursing the woman who got her baby back. Even she wasn't alone...or guilty for that matter. The sister paid the pool boy to pull off the kidnapping. Can't believe I didn't see that coming.

As the credits rolled, I glanced at the clock on the wall and realized that I was less than a half-hour away from the finish line. I looked up at the bags on my IV stand. They were almost empty.

*Just a few more minutes.*

—

No one at the hospital knew my story. My regular infusion nurses—the ones who had taken care of me the whole time—weren't there. There was no "Huzzah!" for my last treatment. There were no hugs. No high fives. No, "Way to go, Danno!" There was only a simple removal of the needle from my porta-cath and a courteous "Have a nice day."

I walked out of the room and shuffled slowly down the hall. When I reached the elevator, I turned around and looked behind me. At the room. At my journey. Maybe it was the chemo-head. Maybe it was the enormity of being done. Maybe it was the symbolism of the moment. Whatever it was, it begged only one question:

*What the hell just happened?*

---

"Why does this one look so much bigger than the others?" I asked out loud, even though I was the only one present.

I had driven myself to the pharmacy while in the throes of the crap that was my life at the moment and picked up my last five shots of Neupogen. My regular pharmacy didn't have them in stock, so I had to go to a different location. *No big deal,* I thought.

Fool.

I got home, headed to the upstairs bathroom, and opened the bag. I knew the routine.

But this time, the needles looked…bigger. Much bigger. Like, as thick as tennis racquet string bigger.

*Michael. Foxtrotter.*

## 19: BARTENDER! ONE MORE ROUND!

As I took the first needle out of the packaging and prepared to stab it into my thigh, I concluded that despite all that I had endured, this might be the worst part of my day.

As it turned out, I was right. Over the previous four months, I had been skewered by more needles than I could count. None of them felt like this. This one actually drew blood. And because the opening on the needle was bigger, I had to push the medicine in even more slowly than usual, just so my thigh wouldn't burst into flames.

So not only were the needles twice as big—at least—but each injection took twice as long. I told Stephanie, and she was horrified.

"That is so wrong. You have to take those back."

"They're too expensive," I said.

"But you can't keep going through this!"

"It's only a minute a day. I'll be fine."

And with that, I cemented my bravery into her DNA. She wanted me bad. At least, that's what I told myself.

Damn chemo-head.

Over the next three days, the nastiness of the side effects began to subside. Even the shots became a little easier. Yes, they still sucked hard, but if that was the worst part of my day, then my days were definitely getting better.

On the last day, for the last shot, I decided to do something grandiose in celebration: I would turn the bag upside-down and let the last syringe fall into my hand.

It felt grandiose at the time.

Wearing boxers and basking in the glory of a final self-impalement, I sat on the toilet lid and upended the bag. Out fell the syringe, right into the palm of my hand. And then, something else fell out of the bag. Do you know what that something else was?

A packet of adapters to make the needles smaller.

I was a moron. A giant, perforated moron. As penance for my idiocy, I shunned the adapters and jammed the final big needle straight into my thigh. I felt I deserved it. It was my way of saying, "Cancer, you didn't beat me up quite enough. Here, let me help you."

To this day, I don't know which was stupider: not looking in the bag or not using what was in the bag once I did.

Good riddance, cancer. You bastard.

# 20
## THE PET SCAN

"The latest scan…shows…" Dr. Needles announced.

"Go on," I nudged. We were on pins and needles.

"…you have no discernable trace of cancer in your body."

"Yes!" I shrieked, hugging the small army in the room—my mom, my dad, my brother, Stephanie, and yes, Dr. Needles. "Thank you so much!"

Apart from the recurring finger tingling, ear ringing, and occasional bouts of constipation, I felt like I could take on the world.

The nausea was gone, and my thinking had cleared to my normal, skewed view of life.

My mother was in tears as my dad held her tight. "Thank God. Thank God," she kept whispering.

"Fucking awesome," my brother concluded.

Stephanie gave me a scritch on the back of my bald head. Life was finally perfect.

"I just want to do one more test to confirm," said Dr. Needles.

"Anything you need," I said, figuring it was a blood test or something equally trivial.

"It's brand new. It's called a PET scan, and it's pretty amazing. It will be able to show any clusters of cancer cells in the body," said Dr. Needles.

"That's awesome!" I said, naïvely.

"It takes about an hour. You can do it right here in the hospital. You'll come in, you'll be catheterized, and we'll do the test," said Dr. Needles.

"Wait…what?"

"You can do it right here in the hospital."

"No, I understand that. What do you mean catheterized?"

"You know what a cath…"

"Yes, I know what a catheter is. Why is it necessary?"

"To prevent a false positive test."

"Do I have to?"

"Yes."

I took a deep breath. I had never been catheterized, but I'd heard about it. I didn't like the thought of having a thick rubber tube jammed up my urethra, but if this is what it would take, this is what it would take.

"Okay. I'll do what you say."

## 20: THE PET SCAN

—

"Huh."

The orderly lifted my gown to discover something he hadn't banked on. Right after I was born, my parents were advised that lopping the top was not only unnecessary, but also potentially harmful. I don't know who the crackpot doctor was who told them this, but they took his advice.

"What's wrong?" I asked, not encouraged by the look on his face.

"Nothing we can't handle, sir," said the orderly.

He walked across the room to the phone, picked it up, and dialed a three-digit number.

"Hi, it's Mark in radiology. We're going to need an extra pair of hands down here. Thanks."

Extra. Pair. Of. Hands.

"What do you need an extra pair of hands for, sir?"

"One of us will fold the skin back while the other inserts the catheter."

I spiked a fever the moment the words left his lips. Fifty different scenarios of how, exactly, this was going to go popped into my head. None of them had a positive outcome. Sweat poured out of places I didn't know could sweat.

The next thing I knew, a six-five knuckle-dragger tromped through the door and immediately put on a pair of rubber gloves, snapping each finger in the process. With each crack of the rubber against his phalanges, my testicles ascended a tick more.

Mark, if that was indeed Tweedledumb's name, squeezed a transparent jelly onto his gloved finger and made a beeline for my no-no triangle.

"What's that for?" I asked, making a fist with my ass.

"It's numbing gel for the entry point," replied Mark.

I'd never thought about that orifice as an "entry" point. *See*: terror.

"We don't have to do this," I reasoned.

Mark was unmoved, as was the knuckle-dragger.

Wrestlemania ensued. I began inching my body to the top of the bed—almost involuntarily—to put as much distance as I could between myself and these men who came at me with four hands and a rubber hose.

"Relax!" one of them yelled.

"I'm trying!" I yelled back.

After a solid two minutes, they were unable to nail the entry. I'm sure my writhing didn't help. To top it all off—I shit you not—at the height of the bedlam, the knuckle-dragger yelled, "Look, do you want this up there or not?"

"Is this a fucking trick question?" I screamed.

"More lube!" barked Mark to no one in particular. There were only two of them; both of them were covered in lube to their elbows.

It wouldn't have mattered if a tanker full of KY unloaded on my nether regions. It wasn't going to happen in this state of chaos. Thing One and Thing Two backed off and tried a kinder, gentler approach.

"Look, I know this is tough, but we have to do this. Take this," Mark said, handing me a towel, "and bite down and scream as hard as you want. But for this to work, you have to remain still."

## 20: THE PET SCAN

I was nearly in tears, but I knew there was no getting out of this. I bit down on the towel, and the two men, by the grace of God and a tube and a half more lubricant, achieved their goal.

—

A PET scan is like a CT on blow. Cancer cells just love to eat glucose; they feed on it like piranha. For a PET scan, glucose gets pumped through your veins via I.V. If any large, glowing areas show up on the scan, you're hosed. If there are none, you're in the clear. When I signed up for this, I didn't realize there was a door number three.

—

"We're going to have to do it again."

I could tell by the look on Dr. Needles's face that he knew as soon as he uttered those words, I would strangle him, laughing while I did. However, I was too caught off guard to attack.

"Come again?"

"The PET. It was inconclusive."

"What does 'inconclusive' mean?"

"Well, there's a bit of a nebulous area that may or may not be cancerous."

"So, again, what does this mean?"

"It means that we're going to have to do the PET scan again."

The good doctor started perspiring. He had heard about the skirmish with the orderlies, and he knew what he was asking me to do. I had agreed to the first PET, catheter and all, because it was supposed to be *the* definitive test to determine whether or not we had beaten the beast.

A second PET, however, would not happen without some serious modifications.

"You want another PET? Fine. Put me out."

"We can't devote those type of hospital resources just to avoid some mild discomfort."

"Mild discomfort? Are you fucking kidding me?"

He dug in. "Dan, there's no choice."

I dug harder. "Yes there is. Put me out, or I'm not doing it."

"Dan."

"No."

"Danny."

My mom, who was sitting beside me and holding my hand, was caught in an impossible situation. So was my dad. He just looked me in the eye with his strong, stoic gaze.

"I'm not doing it again."

My mother tried reasoning. "But what if you still have cancer?"

"Then I still have it. I'll do more chemo."

You know it's bad when you pick five days of four-hour chemo treatments as the lesser of evils. Dr. Needles was unmoved.

"It doesn't work like that, Dan."

"Then I guess you'll have to find another way. I am now—officially—done."

And with that, I walked out of the room, to my car, and drove away, never once looking back to see if anyone followed me. At that moment, I didn't care.

# 21

## PULLING A JESUS

The full-court-press was on. My dear, sainted mother was frantic.

"Danny, I can't make you do this…but you have to do this."

"No, I don't."

My dad made it more personal.

"Dan, I watched my dad die of cancer. I don't want to see you with him."

That one almost worked. I was close to relenting.

"I'm going to be fine, dad. I promise."

I had no idea if I would be fine. It didn't matter.

Stephanie took a brilliant approach: she saw my point.

"Do I think you should do it? Yes. Will I be mad at you if you don't? No. It was a brutally traumatic experience, and if I were you, I wouldn't want to go through it again, either."

"But you would go through it, wouldn't you?"

"If I had no choice, yes. But no one can live your life for you, but you."

God, I love that woman.

I didn't know what to do. Sure, I'd get another PET scan—but only under the condition that I would not have to endure another catheter. A catheter-less PET scan. That, I could agree to. But how the hell was I supposed to make that happen? For the first time in a long time, I was answerless.

I've always prided myself on finding ways around obstacles. Once, during my second semester at the Vancouver Film School, we were shooting a short film called *Waiting for Jennifer*. Vancouver weather is dicey at best, and on the fourth day of filming, we woke up to a driving rainstorm. We were supposed to shoot outside that day in Queen Elizabeth Park.

We called our pal Rob in the equipment room to ask him his thoughts. He had been a student at VFS himself, so we expected some good advice on wet-weather gear for the camera and microphones.

"You couldn't pay me enough money in the world to shoot in this shit."

Thanks for the advice, *Rob*.

Needless to say, the crew was a tick on the flustered side. This was the first time any of us had encountered an obstacle that stopped us dead in our tracks. Shooting outside was a no-go.

## 21: PULLING A JESUS

Postponing the shoot was out of the question, since we had only six days to film the whole thing, and each day was planned down to the minute. And we couldn't simply cut the scene, because omission would have messed up the flow of the story and dropped us below the minimum time constraint of the finished product. In short, we were screwed.

As we contemplated educational suicide, someone in our crew threw up a Hail Mary: "We could always rewrite the scene, I guess."

The plot of the film was simple enough: a man gives his business card to a woman at a bar the night before and spends the next day "waiting for Jennifer," all the while daydreaming about the possibilities of dating her. The original scene we were supposed to shoot that day was a slow-motion shot of two people running towards each other in the park. They smack into each other and fall down in ecstasy.

Because of the weather, that scene was out. So we took the story indoors, to my apartment, a loft where we had filmed a few earlier scenes. The gear was already there, negating the need for a company move to another location.

The new scene showed our man sleeping naked on his stomach in bed. He rolls over to reveal Jennifer beneath him, also naked. They look at each other, smile, and then reach out of either side of the frame to grab already-lit cigarettes. Simultaneous drag. And cut.

The original scene was funny. The one we devised and directed in response to our meteorological crisis was brilliant. The scene got the biggest laugh in each of its two screenings at the Vancouver International Film Festival. It was the only student film to be admitted that year.

But that was just the life and death of a scene. This was potentially the life and death of me, and I didn't have a clue how to write my way out of it. I knew I needed the test. I didn't know how I could ever rationalize making it happen.

—

Two nights later, I still obsessed over the question. Dr. Needles had called me personally to try to talk me into the PET, but I was utterly opposed. And the harder he pushed, the more I dug in. In fact, I stopped talking to anyone about it and got snippy with anyone who tried to bring it up.

I needed to clear my head, so I met some friends for dinner at Schneithorst's, the place where it all began for Steph and me. I looked good at this point. My hair had started sprouting buds, my weight was almost back to normal, and the diversion of good company really buoyed my spirits. We talked about Stephanie, the engagement, the absurdities of cancer treatment, and what everyone else had been doing with their lives. It was a magical night.

As time marched on, people started leaving, one by one. I knew the end of my respite was in sight, and I stopped talking. Fear gripped me again, and I couldn't shake it. My friends noticed. I deflected the first two questions about what was wrong.

"Nothing," I lied.

But my friends knew me better than I knew myself, and they weren't buying it.

"Don't be an asshole. What's wrong?"

I relayed the story of my original PET, which apparently was one of the funniest things they'd ever heard. Their response did not help my mood.

"And now the bastard wants me to get another one," I said… the bastard being Dr. Needles.

## 21: PULLING A JESUS

"So?" they chorused.

"And who's to say that it will work? It didn't the first time. What if it's just a vicious cycle, over and over? The guy's probably a masochist. You should see the look that he gives me with every new test he orders."

The look on my face must have shocked them into submission; their smiles evaporated. I breathed heavily, and I'm pretty sure my left eye twitched. As far as they were concerned, I had officially gone off the deep end, and they were scared. I regretted unloading on them.

"I'm sorry," I said. "I don't know what to do. And I'm petrified."

For a good thirty seconds, everyone was silent. And then, from left field, "You know, you could just pull a Jesus."

"Excuse me. What?"

"What did Jesus do before he died?"

"He was nailed to a cross," I said.

"Before that."

"He was sentenced to death."

"Before that."

"He was kissed by Judas, that prick."

"Before that."

"He...uh...made a reservation for thirteen?"

"Before that."

"Will you tell me already?" I yelled, thoroughly pissed off at this point.

"He fasted."

"So?"

"So...why do you need a catheter?"

"I don't know...I guess so that there's nothing in my bladder to make a false positive."

"So what would happen if you already had nothing in your bladder?"

To this day, I don't remember which one of my friends made the suggestion. I've asked all of them, and no one remembers saying it. But I know the conversation happened.

*What would Jesus do? He wouldn't have anything to drink after midnight, that's what He would do.*

—

"I'm going to do the PET scan."

Ah, the words Dr. Needles wanted to hear.

"That's great! Let's schedule you this week."

"I'm only doing it on one condition."

Dr. Needles frowned. "What condition?"

"I'm going to fast from any food or water for three days, and I'm doing it without a catheter."

"Dan, I can't do that."

"Why not? Would it medically work?"

Dr. Needles thought for a moment. "I guess it would, but you risk severe dehydration by doing this."

"I'll take dehydration over being catheterized."

He stared at me. "And there's no talking you out of doing this?"

"No."

"You know I can't recommend you do this."

"You didn't."

Stare down. I had already survived one with Nana in Ireland. Compared to her, Dr. Needles was child's play.

"It's up to you," I said. "You want the test. This is *my* body. This is *my* choice."

## 21: PULLING A JESUS

"And there's no catheter?" I asked.

"No," said the orderly.

"You're sure?"

"Yes."

As I gently glided into the machine that looked like the CT on crack, I closed my eyes and smiled, thanking Jesus, Dr. Needles, and my faceless friend, though not necessarily in that order.

# 22

## LOSING LEFTY

I was the only twenty-nine year old male in the waiting room that day, a room occupied with women in various stages of pregnancy. It was time for my third ball-trasound. It's the same test given to pregnant women, only instead of being wanded across the belly, I would get mine up my perineum.

Quite a few women gave me the stink-eye that morning. *What's this icky boy doing here?* their faces seemed to say. I can take only so much self-conscious writhing.

"There's an issue with my testicles," I announced.

No one cracked a smile.

And of course, these were the days before HIPPA, so when the nurse opened the door to call the next patient, she used my first and last name.

"Dan Duffy?"

"He's that guy from *Steve and DC*," I heard one woman murmur.

At this point, I'd had two of these, but because I was in the throes of cancer at the time, I didn't really remember them. This one I would remember vividly.

They brought me into a darkened room with the ultrasound machine, a broom closet for changing into the ass-less gown, soft music, and a vase with a single red rose in the corner. I immediately surveyed the den of seduction. *Please God,* I silently prayed, *don't let the ultrasounder be attractive. Give me someone matronly, paunchy, even a homosexual male. As long as it's not someone screaming hot, I won't have to worry about pitching a pup tent.*

After I had completed my instructions from the nurse, which included getting naked and putting on the gown, I hopped up on the table and lay down on my back.

Here's where it got tricky.

The wanding process is very specific; everything has to be in place for it to be a successful excursion. My gown was pulled up. A strategically placed towel kept my todger out of the way by holding it up and back against my FUPA (Fat Upper Pubic Area). The twins were exposed, but they were riding bareback on another towel, which prevented any jelly from dripping down my inner thighs. For the visual: my only exposed parts were my face, my feet, and my sack.

And then Rosemary came in. She was in her mid-fifties, four-foot-eleven, and sporting blue, thick-rimmed eyeglasses. Her dark

## 22: LOSING LEFTY

hair was pulled back tightly in a bun. She was shaped like the back of a bus, God bless her.

In other words, Rosemary was perfect.

"So why are you here today?" she asked as she sat down next to me.

I told her my cancer story and how Dr. Needles wanted both of the boys checked out to make sure the left side had stopped producing cancer cells and the right one wouldn't try to kill me like his brother did.

Rosemary picked up the goo bottle, shook it, and pointed the nozzle towards the triumvirate. She squeezed the bottle for a good three seconds. Because all jelly is cold, I braced myself for impact. However, this jelly had a new chemical in it that warms up when it touches the skin. I have to say, it was a nice surprise.

I would totally buy this product, were it available at Walgreens. Had Mark and the knuckle-dragger used this originally, we might have had a successful first PET. *Might have.*

What was not a nice surprise was the way Rosemary manipulated the wand like the stick shift in a Lamborghini. A ball-trasound is not the most delicate procedure. I shut my eyes and prayed for it to be over quickly.

"So, has it warmed up outside?"

Seriously, Rosemary? You're going to try to have a conversation with me while I'm in this position? Next time, I would pray for a guy to do this. A guy would understand. A guy would be a little gentler. A guy wouldn't ask, "Have you tried the new oven roasted turkey at Panera? It's to die for!"

But then Rosemary dropped this bomb:

"There's the core on the left. And you have some calcium deposits on the right side."

Calcium deposits, or calcium scarring, is an odd thing when you've had testicular cancer. Doctors aren't quite sure what it means. Fifty percent of them will say it's a natural occurrence. Fifty percent will say it's a precursor to cancer. Whatever glimmer of confirmation the wanding was meant to produce shriveled up and died.

—

"I'm going to keep an eye on the right one on a year-to-year basis," said Dr. Needles.

In a nutshell (no pun intended), this little indignity would be as regular as birthdays or Christmas or a prostate exam after forty. Once a year, I would have to consent to Rosemary—or the entire visiting nurses association—manhandling my testicles.

Or, rather, testicle.

"And we'll have to perform a radical orchiectomy."

At first, I thought he was talking about some kind of Tony Hawk skateboarding trick. I could almost hear the X-Games commentators describing the move:

Commentator 1: "An olly, a front side air…and look at that radical orchiectomy! Whoa! Where'd he pull that out of, Tommy?"

Commentator 2: "From the scrote, Billy!"

"What's a radical orchiectomy?" I asked, not wanting to know the answer.

"We're going to remove your left testicle."

*Shit.*

I'm sure it's always a horrendous experience when you are told you are going to lose a body part, but it almost seems gratuitous

## 22: LOSING LEFTY

and slightly cruel when reproductive organs are in the equation. I was afraid I would no longer feel like a full man.

Before the surgery, Stephanie and I had a long talk. She assured me that she would not think of me differently if I had only one, and I believed her. The one question I still had, however, was if she still wanted to be with me. I had known too many people who fall in love and get married thinking life is going to be a certain way, and when it's not, they find themselves in a mess of trouble.

"You know I'm losing lefty," I said.

"Yes," she replied. "And it doesn't make a difference to me."

"Well, it might. You know I went to the sperm bank the day after I started, and it might not work."

"I'm not worried."

"But what if we can't have kids? I know you want kids."

"I want you. Kids are just a bonus. I said 'yes' to you."

Her words made me 95% okay with saying goodbye to the little shit that tried to kill me. The other 5% of okay came from an unlikely source.

Steve and DC had asked me to visit their show and tell my story to listeners who had followed my call-in updates every few weeks. My good friend Traci was an afternoon jock on our sister radio station, The Point. After I chatted with the *Steve and DC* crew, I went down the hall to visit Traci, whom I hadn't seen since I'd been diagnosed.

The second I walked into the room, she gave me a big hug and asked how I was. I told her that life was basically amazing, Steph and I were happy and in love, and I was almost done with my treatment, except for one last biggie.

"What's the biggie?" she asked.

"They're taking lefty tomorrow."

Without missing a beat, she gave me this pearl of wisdom: "Ya know, Danno, sometimes a guy just doesn't want a roommate."

At that moment, I was finally ready to say goodbye. No tears would be shed, no memories would be held tight, no sadness would be felt. A body part is just a body part, and being short a testicle wasn't going to make me any less of a man than a mastectomy makes a woman any less of a woman or the loss of a leg makes anyone less of a runner or the loss of an organ makes anyone less human. We are not the sum of our parts. We are what is in our hearts and our souls. And I was content that good things filled mine.

*Adios, huevo.*

---

"What are we doing today?"

Dr. Leonard Gaum was my urologist. He had a Saharan wit and the bedside manner of Bill Belichick with sleep apnea. But he was the best of the best, and therefore worth the hassle.

"Uh...radical orchiectomy."

"Which side?"

"The left," I said.

"Are you sure?" he asked.

"What do you mean am I sure? Am I wrong?"

"No."

"Then why did you ask?"

"I had to be sure you were sure."

I managed to fire off a "What the hell?" before I passed out.

# 23

## THE MIRACLES

"So I've got bad news, more bad news, and good news." I had missed Dr. Leonard Gaum's wit, something I hadn't experienced in quite a while. Stephanie and I had been happily married for a year and a half, and it was time to start building a family. We were not going to adopt a child. Adoption is truly amazing and a real gift to all involved, but it didn't feel like the right thing for us. And because I hadn't been able to release the hounds before I started chemo, we didn't have a good feeling about IVF.

We said that if we couldn't have children, we would move to New York, our favorite city on Earth. Steph would be a pharmacist, and I would produce videos. And we would live happily ever after. But before we loaded up the truck and moved to a deluxe apartment in the sky, I would get tested to see if we even could have children the non-IVF way. This meant a return visit to my urologist extraordinaire, Dr. Gaum.

I had to go through the exact same drill as I did when I failed so epically with Nurse Ratchet, bad porn, and the sterile cup. But this time I brought my own magazine, which I had purchased on the way to the event and donated to the cause upon exit. What took twenty-six minutes and caused welts last time took all of four minutes this time. Three days later, the results were ready.

"What's the first bad news?" I asked.

"A third of your sperm are dormant."

"Meaning?"

"Dead."

"Great."

"The second piece of bad news is that a third of your sperm are deformed."

"Deformed?"

"Picture a boat without a rudder."

"So they're..."

"Useless."

"Marvelous."

"The good news is—and frankly I can't explain it considering the amount of chemotherapy you had—a third have survived and appear healthy and intact."

"Really? Meaning..."

## 23: THE MIRACLES

"Meaning, there's no medical reason I see why you can't have children the natural way."

I was stunned. Never in my wildest dreams did I think we had a shot at having children naturally.

"Now go practice, young man."

Dr. Gaum gave me a wink and a hint of a smile.

Five seconds. Mind blown...twice.

—

"There's something wrong with this wine."

Stephanie and I and twelve of our closest friends were enjoying an evening at our favorite little spot, Brennan's, in the Central West End neighborhood of St. Louis. Stephanie was not a fan of the merlot I had chosen.

"Are you okay?" I asked.

She leaned forward. "This wine is making me sick to my stomach."

"May I have yours then?"

Smack.

—

"Are you ready? Bear is about to dook himself."

I stood at the top of the stairs, leash in hand. Bear, our Aussie Cattle Dog mix, was beside himself at his good fortune. It was a Friday in late May, and both Steph and I had taken the day off. The morning was sunny and slightly crisp, perfect walking weather. Stephanie came out from the bedroom.

"Ready," she smiled. "Bear! Are we goin' for a walk?"

Sixty-three pounds of Bear dragged me down the stairs. He's a strong little bugger. As I regained my bearings at the bottom, I looked behind me to say something to Steph. She wasn't there.

"Babe?"

"You need to come up here."

I could hear in her voice she was crying. I dropped the leash and raced upstairs.

"Where are you?"

"The bathroom."

I walked in to find her holding the pregnancy test she had taken twenty minutes earlier, our third since my visit with Dr. Gaum.

"What do two pink lines mean?" I asked.

"It means that I know why I can't stomach wine lately."

"So you're not allergic?"

"No." Stephanie smiled through her tears. "Thank God."

—

"Did I just pee myself?" Stephanie asked, shifting on the couch where we sat watching the news.

It was Thursday night, February 9, 2006. We had been spoiling ourselves over the past few days, our last as just a cute couple with a dog. We were mired in a food coma from Yen Ching, our second favorite Chinese restaurant on planet Earth. Really good beef curry.

"I don't know, did you?"

"My undies are a little wet."

"You want me to get you a fresh pair?"

Half an hour later, while lying in bed and watching a re-run of *Seinfeld*, Stephanie squirmed.

"Oh no," she said. "I did it again."

## 23: THE MIRACLES

"Do you want me to get you another pair?" I asked.
"You better get my phone. I think my water just broke."

—

"C'mon, kid. C'mon!"
One minute, Stephanie was trying to push out our baby. The next, she was being wheeled out of the room and into surgery for an emergency cesarean. Dr. Kent Branson, her amazing OB-GYN, was in a race to save our son's life.

Stephanie's labor began the natural way, plus epidural. However, her hips were not very wide, and our baby was now stuck in the birth canal.

I held her hand the entire time, keeping her calm, looking into her eyes, assuring her that everything was going to be fine. In reality, my heart was in my throat.

Dr. Branson was trying to pry the tiny head out of the birth canal, but it was wedged so tightly.

"C'mon kid!"

Stephanie started crying as if she had somehow done something wrong. Of course, she hadn't. I'd never met such a doting mother-to-be. She constantly read out loud to him, she ate healthy things, and she exercised throughout her entire pregnancy, including yesterday morning at the YMCA.

Yet here we were, fighting for our sanity as our little one fought for his life.

"That's it. That's it! Keep comin', kid!"

Stephanie and I held our breath. As distressed as I was, I couldn't begin to imagine what she was going through. Sympathy and empathy are two vastly different things.

And then, we heard it. The faint cry of a newborn baby. Samuel Alaric Duffy came into the world on the afternoon of Friday, February 10, 2006. He was seven pounds and one ounce of perfection. As soon as I saw him, a voice from that chilly October night I almost died on an interstate echoed in my head.

"You're here for a reason, kid."

—

"Did you feel that?" Stephanie asked as I stepped out of the shower.

"Feel what?" I asked.

"The earthquake."

"Excuse me?"

On the morning of April 18, 2008, at 4:37 a.m., a 5.4-magnitude earthquake rocked the southern part of Illinois, not far from where we lived in Missouri. For some reason—perhaps it was the shower or perhaps I was simply not paying attention—I didn't feel a thing.

I learned later that the earthquake was strong enough to topple chimneys in South St. Louis and crumble a small part of a concrete viaduct. Tremors were felt as far away as Atlanta, Georgia.

"He's coming in with a bang," I said.

*He* was our second son, Benjamin August Duffy, who came into the world via planned C-section by Dr. Kent Branson, M f-ing D. For obvious reasons, Stephanie and I didn't want to risk a second natural birth attempt.

"Oh, you'll love it," said Dr. Branson. "You can get your hair done the day before, pre-pack your bags, eat whatever you want for dinner, show up the next morning, and *poof*. Baby."

## 23: THE MIRACLES

True to form, the good doc was right on the money. Everything went off without a hitch. Well, almost everything. I got yelled at by a nurse for breaking the sterile field.

"Mr. Duffy, if you do that again, I will have to ask you to leave!" I swear I heard Dr. Branson laughing at me.

But I did learn a valuable lesson from the experience: it is better to ask forgiveness than permission.

I had been taking pictures in the delivery room because I was prepared, dammit. All of a sudden, Dr. Branson spits out, "There's his head!" Immediately, I reached my hand over the drape and snapped a picture. In hindsight, I probably should have turned off the flash, but, hey...no one's perfect. This is, of course, when I got yelled at. And I did feel bad about breaking protocol. Until I saw the picture. It was nothing short of miraculous.

Unable to see what I was shooting, I snapped the shot of a lifetime. Our son's head had emerged from Stephanie's belly, the only part of his body now in the outside world, and his face looked right at the camera lens. If you paid me a million dollars to plan a shot like that, I still couldn't capture the moment I managed to steal virtually blindfolded. As my friend Teri says, "That's God winking at you."

When the nurses toweled him off and laid him on the scale for weight and height, I couldn't help but notice how...big...he was.

"How does he look?" Stephanie asked.

"Gifted."

In the midst of all the chaotic love and admiration that surrounds childbirth, the voice visited my thoughts once more: "You're here for a reason, kid."

# 24

## IT CAN'T BE DONE

The birth of my children irreversibly changed me. When I call them my miracle boys, I'm not kidding. Some people with perfect plumbing still have issues conceiving. Yet here I was, running at half capacity, with only a third of that half functioning at all, and I fathered two beautiful sons.

As far as I was concerned, Stephanie, Sam and Ben—and even Bear—were gifts straight from God, and it was high time I thanked Him for them. My issue: I didn't have a clue where to start.

One night not long after Benjamin was born, some friends and I were eating dinner at Schneithorst's. (Yes, it always goes back to Schneithorst's.) Our friend David had just directed his first feature, and we were all itching to make movies and score deals and become gazillionaires.

"What we need are some compelling stories," said Joe, the man who produced David's film.

"I could do nudity," said Richard to no one in particular.

"Stories are the hard part," said our friend, Scott. "Once you have those, the rest is easy."

"Well, I've kinda wanted to tell my own story about cancer. Just how insane it was. And I want to see if I can help others avoid the same shit I fell into. So," I paused, "I could try writing a script, I guess."

Other than a few non-fiction video projects, I had never written anything narrative but a short film script, and I'd certainly never written one with any kind of substance.

Scott, who works for a very large and very famous production company in LA, gave me a nudge.

"Give it a shot. I'd love to see what you can do."

"How long do you want it?" I asked.

"If you can write a hundred pages in script format, that would work."

*A hundred pages?* I thought. *Is he serious? I've never written anything that long in my life. I'll never fill a hundred pages!*

———

One hundred and eighty-six pages later, I had written my first script. When I handed a copy to each of the guys, I got the same response:

"You want us to read all this?"

And when they handed me their notes on my script, I wondered if a couple of the guys planned on using a few pages when they ran out of Charmin. Nestled in the criticism, however, was the boost I needed:

*Keep writing.*

It's one thing when people tell you that you're absolutely no good at something. But it's quite another when they give you even a nugget of hope: "You know, this blows, but there's an idea or two in there that may be worth saving."

So for the better part of eighteen months, I wrote. And wrote. And wrote. I tweaked here, trimmed there, blew up the entire script twice, and re-wrote every rewrite of my previous rewrites.

When I felt that I had really written the story I wanted to tell, I shared it with a few people. Joe, the man who produced David's film, was the first. His thoughts: "It doesn't completely suck."

Score!

Then I shared it with my friend Craig, one of my former instructors from film school and, currently, the lead cinematographer for one of the most successful franchises on television. His thoughts: "I've never really seen anything like this. I'd love to shoot it for you."

I met a new friend online named Maneli. Someone shared a YouTube video of him, and I thought he was the most gifted guitarist I'd ever seen. I reached out to him and sent him a copy of the script, asking him if he'd be willing to write some music for the movie. After reading it, he told me he loved it and he'd be willing to record some songs for it on the cheap, and possibly even play a fundraiser for it.

I also shared it with Karen, a casting director in Hollywood. Her thoughts: "This is awesome. It has so much heart. Get some dough in the bank, and you won't believe who I can get for you."

And therein lies the rub. Movies are expensive. I was relatively poor. How would I even attempt to get this thing made?

---

"We need a name."

I recruited Joe to help me turn the script into a film. He had done a fantastic job with David's film, and I wanted his expertise. Joe is also a realist, meaning he would keep me grounded or at least inspire me to prove him wrong.

And Joe was absolutely right. Without major connections to get funding, we needed someone who could help us raise money. Perhaps, we thought, a well-established charity might be the way to go. And maybe, in return, we could give them a chunk of the profits for their mission.

"Who's got a name?" I asked.

"There's Livestrong. Or maybe the American Cancer Society? Those are the two biggies," Joe suggested.

"Let's try American Cancer," I said. "Maybe we can start with the local office."

"Good idea."

---

"American Cancer Society, this is April." April was the director of communications for the ACS of Eastern Missouri.

## 24: IT CAN'T BE DONE

"Hi, April, my name is Dan Duffy, and I'm a local filmmaker in St. Louis."

"Hi, how can I help you?"

*She wants to help us! We're off to a good start!*

"Well, we're thinking of trying to raise money to make a film about a man with cancer, and we wanted to see if, maybe, you'd be willing to partner with us. In return, we would share some of the profits with you."

"Huh. That's interesting, but we've really never done that sort of thing."

*Dang it. Stonewalled.*

"Is there anyone there who might be willing to talk with us?" I asked.

"Tell you what…can you send me something in writing? An e-mail, maybe?"

*Door cracked.*

"I'll be happy to. Thank you!"

We exchanged e-mail addresses, and I got to work. The idea was simple: we raise money, the American Cancer Society lets us use their name to help raise the money, and we give them a portion of all profits. I also gussied up the e-mail with both Joe's and my accomplishments. *We were serious filmmakers,* I wrote, *and we were serious about getting this film made.*

I re-read my letter a few dozen times and hit send. It was 2:15 p.m.

At 4:15 p.m., as I stood in line at the grocery store, my phone rang. The first three digits matched April's phone number at the ACS.

"Hello?"

"Hi, Dan, it's April from the American Cancer Society."

"Hi, April! Did you get my e-mail?"

"Oh, we're going way bigger than that."

*Door kicked in.*

"I read it and thought it had merit, so I sent it to division, which is our regional office. They read it and thought it had merit, so they've sent it to national. And now Angela from national wants to talk to you."

*Oh, my God.*

"April, you got us through the entire bureaucracy of the American Cancer Society in two hours?"

"Nope. You did."

—

"Okay, you're a go."

Joe and I sat in my small office, sweating profusely. We were on one end of the conference call, while the heads of the American Cancer Society's marketing team sat in their conference room on the other end of the call. For forty-five minutes, we told them our story. They asked us a ton of questions, and we gave them straight answers. Apparently, we impressed them. Not only did they give us permission to use their name and logo to solicit funds for the movie, but they would also help us market it once it was made.

Then we tried to take it one step too far.

"Would you be willing to host a fundraising effort for us so that we can ask for tax-free donations?"

"Well, that's a bit of a gray area," said the head of the marketing team. "Because you don't actually work for us, it would essentially be a call to action, and you'd be taxed on it. So, if you needed seven hundred thousand to make the film, you'd have to raise over a million. What you should do is start your own non-profit."

*Door slammed.*

After the phone call ended, Joe and I looked at each other and laughed.

"Yeah, like that's ever gonna happen," I said.

"Not a chance," he agreed.

—

"Why am I seeing you today?"

Joann was as no-nonsense a lawyer as they come, which is saying something, but no one in the Midwest knew more about not-for-profit law. When she saw two thirty-something guys walk into her office, we must have given off the sweet smell of failure. She didn't appear all that thrilled to see us. I couldn't imagine why.

What Joann hadn't yet realized was that my desire to help other people with cancer through this film had slowly woven its way into my being and had become, in essence, part of my DNA. Three minutes into the conversation, when she saw just how serious we were, she cracked a smile.

*We've got her,* Joe and I thought.

And then, God winked again. Over the next fifty minutes, the skeleton and guts of a mission were born. The name would be The Half Fund. The mission would be not only to make our own film but also to perpetuate the creation of commercial art—movies or books or music or documentaries—that would educate people about cancer.

We would make the first film. Half the profits would go to the American Cancer Society. The other half would be fed back into The Half Fund, which would give the money to other artists to work on more projects. Those artists would then split their profits, half to the cancer charity of their choice and half to us. In this way, The Half Fund would be completely self-regenerating.

"I know of nothing else like this," said Joann, "but I think you have a shot. Be very, very specific in your application, give me the meat, and I'll fill in the rest."

And that's exactly what we did, and that's exactly what she did. In our application, we tried to think of every single question an IRS agent would ask—usage, motives, anything. And once we asked the questions of ourselves, we put the answers into final form. Joann was impressed. She filled in the legalese, and we were ready to submit.

"Good luck, gentlemen. I think you've really got something here. Prepare to answer a few questions if you get a positive response, and if you are religious, pray for an agent who's been affected by cancer. Because what you're doing has never been done before. And it's hard to get passage without a precedent."

---

Almost nine months to the day later, a letter came from the Internal Revenue Service. It was addressed to The Half Fund.

*We are pleased to inform you that upon review of your application for tax exempt status, we have determined that you are exempt from Federal income tax under section 501(c)(3) of the Internal Revenue Code. You are also qualified to receive tax deductible bequests, devises, transfers, or gifts under section 2055, 2106, or 2522 of the Code. Because this letter could help resolve any questions regarding your exempt status, you should keep it in your permanent records.*

Neither Joe, nor Jo, nor I could quite believe the news.

# 25

## HAITI

Ideas are one thing. Planning and execution are quite another. Whenever Joe and I told people about The Half Fund, they'd respond the same way: "Wow."

One time, we ended up stalking Kevin Smith, the writer and director of *Clerks*, *Mallrats*, *Chasing Amy*, and *Dogma*, among other films. Kevin was an alumnus of the Vancouver Film School and one of the reasons I eventually chose the school for myself. He was taking his latest film, *Red State*, on a cross-country road trip. The closest he would get to St. Louis was Chicago.

"Let's get to him," I told Joe.

Of course, saying you're going to get to someone and actually getting to that someone are two totally different things. We needed a plan.

Kevin's online presence is called the Askewniverse, named after his company, View Askew Productions. One of the main aspects of the website is a message board. Kevin, himself, makes comments on the board, and the diehard fans are very protective of him. Try to get him to do something for you, and they'll make you wish you'd never heard of the *Jersey Trilogy*.

Despite the potentially hostile environment, I started a thread called "A Note to Kevin Smith." I wrote about The Half Fund, what we were doing, and how we wanted to see if he'd be willing to share our mission with others.

I expected major backlash the moment I hit send. Instead, we received the diametric opposite.

"Fucking great idea!"

"That is badass!"

"Good fucking luck with all your endeavors!"

The comments came flooding in. (Askewnivites like to cuss a lot, as does Mr. Smith.)

And then someone wrote this: "You need to get a hold of Jon Gordon, his producer. Here's his Twitter handle."

*Did that just happen?*

That evening, the night before the Chicago showing of *Red State*, I fired off a Tweet to Mr. Gordon, even though I had no idea who he was. My Tweet simply stated, "We hear you're the man to talk with." And I shared the link to the thread from the View Askew message board.

And then I fell asleep.

## 25: HAITI

The next day, Joe and I drove almost five hours from St. Louis to Chicago. As we were pulling in, I checked the message board for any new replies.

"Holy shit!" one of the comments read. "Gordon replied! Good luck!"

*What the...?*

Sure enough, Mr. Gordon had replied to our Tweet.

"@thehalffund...wow...let's talk."

*Really?*

Joe and I made it to our hotel room. As I paced the floor, trying to formulate what I was going to say to Mr. Gordon, Joe popped open his laptop.

"Holy shit. Do you want to know who this guy is?" he asked.

"Oh, hell no," I said.

If I didn't know who Jon Gordon was, I would have no need to fear Jon Gordon. And as far as I knew, he only produced *Red State*. That's the way it was going to stay.

After dinner at Lawry's (fantastic prime rib, by the way), Joe and I walked to the Harris Theater. The show was going to start in thirty-five minutes. A wave of panic washed over my entire body as we walked into the lobby.

"Joe, there's no way they're going to let us backstage."

Thank God my partner was cool under pressure.

"We gotta find someone in the band."

We scanned the room looking for our *in*. Then, we spotted them. Smack dab in the middle of everything, three twenty-something stoner dudes were selling merchandise.

"That's our best bet right there," said Joe.

Thirty seconds later, I stood face to face with the gatekeeper. He was young, blonde, and pierced.

"Is Jon Gordon here?" I asked sheepishly.

"Yeah! Let me get him." And the dude rushed off.

I turned around and looked at Joe.

*Holy shit! Did you see what just happened?*

Two minutes later, Joe and I met Jon Gordon.

"Man, I saw the thread, and I asked Kev about it last night. He thought it was amazing."

This man, a man who would go on to win an Oscar for producing *Silver Linings Playbook* and then be nominated the very next year for *American Hustle*, just told us that he thought our idea was amazing. So did Kevin Smith, perhaps my greatest cinematic influence. I felt a tingle in my special place.

By the end of the conversation, we did as all fathers do: we talked about our children. It was one of the most beautifully surreal moments of my life. To this day, I still send Jon an e-mail around Oscar time, wishing him well. To this day, he always responds.

So not only did our friends and family support us, not only did the American Cancer Society support us, but some of Hollywood's biggest heavyweights supported us. And they all said the same thing: "Wow."

The problem was turning "wow" into dollars. I knew how to tell stories. Joe knew how to put them on a screen. We did not know how to fundraise. At least, we weren't very good at it. Apart from a couple of small events, we were treading water.

Two years into The Half Fund's existence, we had raised a total of twenty thousand dollars. It was enough to cover our expenses and keep a small reserve in the bank, but it was never going to get us where we needed to go. Many times, I questioned whether or not we were on the right track. Other times, I wondered if we were making a difference at all. Were we changing anyone's life? Should we just pack up and call it a day?

At the height of my doubt, a random and unexpected series of events suggested that maybe, just maybe, we weren't wasting our time after all.

I used to work at the radio station with a man named Todd Newton. Todd has since gone on to host *Family Game Night*, *Monopoly Millionaires Club, and The Price is Right* touring show, make countless personal appearances, and give talks around the world.

Todd was coming to town, and he needed a small appearance filmed. My fledgling little video production company had just switched over to high-definition, and I needed to test my camera. I agreed to do it for him, gratis.

The conditions that night were a disaster. The lighting, which was not in our control, was beyond awful. It was so dark, we could barely see anything. And as if that weren't bad enough, a monsoon ensured that only a handful of the sellout crowd actually attended.

"Is it even worth going on?" Todd asked, backstage.

"Let's just shoot it anyway, and I'll see what I can come up with."

The final video was nothing short of a Christmas miracle—and nothing like the actual night. A crowd of hundreds saw Todd pull off an amazing display of talent, with some of the cleanest lighting you've ever seen. He almost fell off the couch when he saw the results. He thanked me, and then we didn't speak again for three months.

Then one day in late September, I got a phone call.

"Hello?"

"Danny, it's Todd Newton."

"Hey, Todd! How are you?"

"I'm great, sir. Hey, how'd you like to go to Haiti?"

*Wait, what?*

Todd had teamed up with an organization called Soles4Souls and was now their goodwill ambassador. He was going to Haiti in early January with the founder, a man named Wayne Elsey. Wayne wanted some footage shot in Port au Prince, and he asked Todd if he knew of anyone who could film it well…and inexpensively.

"Wayne, I know just the guy."

Wayne Elsey was a shoe executive who had a way of treating people the way they needed to be treated at any given time. Once while working at a local shoe store, a group of ladies walked in on a shopping spree. One of the ladies was quite tall, wearing shoes that might have been made by Xerox. As Wayne took all of their measurements, he saw what amounted to shame from the tall woman. As far as she was concerned, her feet were the size of canoes.

Wayne ran to the back and grabbed their sizes. When he returned, he handed each woman a box. For the tall woman, he had placed her shoes in a box that read "8 ½." She almost cried with gratitude. To her, he was a saint. To those who know him, he was being Wayne.

On December 26, 2004, he was sitting on the couch at his home in Orlando when he saw what the rest of us saw that day: the absolute devastation unfolding live off the coast of Thailand. A three-story wall of water slammed into the shore, annihilating everything in its path.

As Wayne sat there, barely able to blink at what he was watching, he saw a single child's shoe wash up on the beach.

*I can do something about that,* he thought.

The next day, as he described it, "I got off the couch and did something." He called his friends in the shoe industry. Two months later, two hundred and fifty thousand pairs of shoes were shipped to the affected area. Then, he went back to work, thinking his good deed was done.

Then came Hurricane Katrina, a disaster—and subsequent need—in his own backyard. Taking his position and the surrounding circumstances as a sign from God, he left the shoe business to start a mission that would help those who didn't have any shoes at all. Soles4Souls was born.

Wayne and I saw a lot of similarities in each other. It's why we were both in Haiti: he to help a country still reeling from a powerful earthquake two years earlier and me to help him tell the Soles4Souls story for nothing more than room, board, and meals.

One day, after I finished interviewing him for a shot in the middle of a street market in Port-au-Prince, I turned off the camera and asked, "Do you think it's weird at all for me, who co-founded a tiny little charitable mission, to help you, who founded a wildly successful charitable mission? Aren't we somehow competing for donor dollars?"

"Dan, you're not my competition. Even other shoe organizations are not my competition. Right now, there are over 280,000,000 kids without a single pair of shoes. My only competition is time."

I understood what he meant with every fiber of my being. Time is precious, fleeting, and you never know how much or little you're going to get. We both understood the importance of doing good with the time we had left.

—

"Hello?"
"Danny, it's Wayne."

I had not talked Wayne in the three months since returning from Haiti.

"How are you, sir?"

"I'm good, buddy. Hey, I wanted to tell you that I'm leaving Soles4Souls to start a new venture to help small organizations like yourselves. What can I do for you?"

One month later, Joe and I flew down to Orlando to meet with Wayne. He gave us a place to stay, he bought us lunch, and he tendered some invaluable advice. We hired him to build a new website for us, as well as to re-brand everything, from logo to mission statement. It was the best money we ever spent.

---

*We'd love to invite you to become a HuffPost blogger! We're hoping you'll add your voice to the mix! Our readers will benefit greatly from your expertise and perspective.*

A member of the Huffington Post blog team read a blog on our website, the website built and designed by the team of Wayne Elsey. We were about to discover a new way to help people devastated by cancer.

# 26

## THE ACCIDENTAL ACTIVIST

"I really needed to read that."

"This helped me so much."

"It's like you reached into my brain and pulled out everything I was feeling."

Joe and I were shocked and humbled to learn that our Huffington Post blogs were affecting people the way they did. With every blog published, new people read our message. I discovered that while we were still far from raising enough funds for the film, we were still fulfilling our mandate to lift the veil on cancer through storytelling.

The blogs facilitated another unexpected result: once people knew that we were completely unafraid to talk about the realities of cancer, they were emboldened to reach out to us. Sometimes it was as simple as a private Facebook message asking for a prayer. Other times, budding bloggers would ask us to read their material and help them find their voice. My friend Chris, the one who was completely unafraid to talk with me about my own cancer, learned of a friend who worked for his family's restaurant who had recently been diagnosed with testicular cancer. Chris wanted to reach out to him, but he didn't quite know what to say. I told him that I would be happy to be an intermediary.

We were finally making a difference, and that difference led to one of the most amazing and unexpected opportunities of my life.

It was the Saturday before Father's Day of 2013. Stephanie and the boys were in the kitchen making me breakfast. They came up the stairs carrying a lovely spread and singing, "Happy Father's Day to you...Cha! Cha! Chocolate!"

After kisses galore, Stephanie said, "Your phone rang while I was downstairs."

No one calls our house before 7:00 a.m., so I excused myself to make sure nothing was wrong with my parents or my brother. I hit the voicemail button.

"Danny, it's Wayne. Give me a call when you get this."

I called him back immediately.

"Hi, Wayne."

"How are ya, pal?"

"I'm great. What's up?"

Wayne had an idea to connect The Half Fund with another fierce cancer advocate, author and all around badass Dr. Sheri Prentiss, and he wanted my thoughts. I wholeheartedly agreed.

"That's great, buddy," Wayne said. "Well, listen, I have to get going. I'm on my way to Sarasota."

"Oh, awesome. Father's day vacation?"

"No, I'm meeting with a lady named Judy to talk about giving a TED talk in October."

If you've never seen a TED talk, their motto is "Ideas Worth Spreading." The talks are limited to eighteen minutes or less, and people like Bill Gates, Steve Jobs, Madeline Albright, and Jeff Bezos have given them all over the world. Wayne was now in discussion to give his own.

"Wayne, let me know where, let me know when, and I will be the loudest cheerer in the audience."

—

"Hi, Judy! Meet Dan Duffy, the man I told you about earlier today about giving a possible TED talk."

I didn't quite believe the e-mail that popped up on my phone as I stood in Stephanie's parents' kitchen. We were in Effingham to celebrate Father's Day with her family. I read it again. And again. And again.

Wayne attended the meeting with Judy, the director of TEDx Sarasota, and realized that he wouldn't be a good fit for giving a talk at the moment. But he told her about three possible speaking candidates for the upcoming event.

I was one of them.

*Holy shit.*

—

"I'm going to pair you with an amazing coach."

Judy had my back from the word go. She knew that I had zero experience speaking in front of a live audience, let alone one at a TEDx event. Still, she believed I could do it.

"I want to give you some help, though."

Help came in the form of Jerry, an audio engineer and producer who has worked with some huge names on some huge projects, including Rod Stewart's "Unplugged" CD. An Orlando native, he volunteered his time to help speakers at TEDx Sarasota that year. His wife, Kathy, was a film producer. Judy believed the three of us would hit it off. She could not have been more right.

Jerry and I talked a few times leading up to the event. He gave me some incredible advice, showing me how to add here and trim there to polish my talk. He walked me through the entire process of writing my eleven-minute monologue, and he gave me the confidence to go beyond myself in ways I never had the courage to do before.

The one thing that plagued me, however, was the finale. Namely, I didn't know how to end it. In my *Steve and DC* days, we were taught to "hook 'em with a headline and leave 'em with a bang." I didn't have my bang, and I couldn't figure out how to find it.

God winked at me one more time.

I sat in my office one morning editing a video project when my phone rang. It was Richard.

"Hello, tart," I said.

Richard was not in the mood to gab. Without so much as a "What's up, trollop," he asked if he could borrow my video camera.

"Sure, what's going on?"

"I have a friend named Deb, and Deb is about to die."

I felt like I'd been kicked in the ball.

# 26: THE ACCIDENTAL ACTIVIST

About six years ago, Deb was taking a shower when she felt a mass in her breast. Because she was a delivery nurse at a local hospital, she was able to finagle a mammogram just three days later. By the look on the radiologist's face after the test, she knew things were very, very bad. Deb had advanced breast cancer. A bi-lateral mastectomy was followed by heavy doses of chemotherapy and radiation.

Thankfully, the treatment seemed to work. After a grueling struggle, she was finally deemed cancer free.

A few months later, the cancer returned. But it didn't come back in her breast tissue; it came back in her brain.

And she beat it.

And then it came back in her lungs.

And she beat it.

And then it came back in her bones.

And she beat it.

And then it came back in her spine.

And she beat it.

And then it came back in her brain.

Again.

This time, though, the treatment didn't work. The cancer progressed. The drugs made her bloated. She had a tumor on her optic nerve that blinded her in one eye and caused it to shut. Because of the former cancer in her legs and in her spine, she was unable to walk. She was always hot. She was always tired. She was, for lack of a better word, trapped in a futile fight.

Yet fight she would, just not for herself. Aware of the short time she had left, she gave her daughter Abby memories that she could carry with her for the rest of her life. They celebrated Christmas on August 28—tree, presents, eggnog, and all.

One day, Abby asked her mom if she was going to make it to her birthday in February. Deb said that it didn't look like it would happen. So they celebrated Abby's birthday early.

And now Richard needed my camera to record Deb, who wanted to say goodbye to her daughter before she was robbed of the ability to do so.

"Do you want me to go with you?" I asked.

"I wouldn't ask that, Danny."

"You didn't, Richard."

Richard and I drove to Deb's house with my camera and audio gear. The sole intention was to let Deb say whatever she was going to say. When we got there, Deb and her pals, Beth and Stacia, greeted us. These ladies were just two of Deb's incredibly close-knit group of friends, the type of friends who would fight with you in the battles of, and for, your life. They were so close that each one had the same Facebook profile picture: all of them together with Deb.

They knew the inevitable. They knew what was in store for them. They refused to run away. They would slap cancer in the face, acknowledging that while it would take Deb's body, it would take neither her soul nor any of theirs. They were some of the bravest people I had ever met.

At first, Deb was reluctant to talk. And she didn't want to be on camera at all.

"It's no problem," I said. "I'll just point the camera elsewhere, and we'll still get what you want to say."

For twenty minutes, she read facts from Abby's baby book: genealogy, time of birth, and so on. Everything seemed very forced. I could tell she was nervous, especially around me. I didn't blame her. She didn't know me from a hole in the wall. And then she said something startling:

"When I found the lump, we met with Dr. Needles."

I had my opening.

"I have to take a break," she said a few minutes later. "Could someone please get me some water?"

While Stacia headed to the kitchen for water, I let slip to Deb, "You know, Dr. Needles was my oncologist, too."

At that moment, everything changed. Once Deb realized she could be herself around me, the books were thrown to the wayside. We started filming again. Her words to her daughter became intensely personal.

I left Deb's house that day knowing that I didn't have much time. She was going to die, and I would do everything in my power to get the footage edited in case she wanted to make any changes.

For the next three days, I sat at my chair editing the most emotionally difficult video I've ever worked on. During the filming, I listened and I didn't listen, because I knew that if I allowed myself to get caught up in the moment, I would have been in worse emotional shape than she was. Now as I watched the footage from the comfort of my edit suite, she blew me away.

She said so many amazing things, but there was one piece of motherly advice that hit me especially hard: "Keep your cool," she said. "I know that this disease has been hard on all of us, kid. And very often, I was not able to keep my cool. And you didn't deserve that. And I'm sorry. So when you're a mommy, please try your best to keep your cool."

As someone who had not always kept his cool with his own children, I bawled when she said this. A torrent of guilt filled every cell in my body, and I vowed to heed her advice.

Then she said something that shoved me over the edge.

"And, Abby, don't forget the pennies from Heaven. Whenever you see a penny, pick it up. That's from me in Heaven. There are going to be signs of me everywhere. I'm not leaving you."

And with that, I sobbed inconsolably. Tears streamed out with a vengeance like I'd never known. I couldn't get it together. I buried my face in my hands and audibly wept. My heart physically hurt.

And at that moment, my phone rang. It was Jerry, wanting to discuss the TEDx talk. I wanted to let it hit voicemail, but Jerry was not the easiest man to get a hold of. I had to take it.

"Hi, Jerry."

"Dan, what's wrong?"

For three solid minutes, I unloaded on this man. Through heavy sobs, I told him everything. How I was so angry at the unfairness of life. How I hated this disease. How I would do everything in my power to take from it what it takes from us.

And when I stopped talking, there was a full minute of silence.

"You there, Jerry?"

"Dan, that's your ending."

---

I made it through the first ten minutes of the TEDx talk without a hitch. The audience laughed at all the laughs, gasped at the picture of my destroyed Jeep, and seemed genuinely interested in my stories of my journey with cancer, my family, The Half Fund, Wayne, and Haiti.

And then, it was Deb's turn. Instead of trying to describe her words, I let her speak for herself. For sixty seconds, the audience heard the voice of a woman who had been given her wings. At one point in the clip, Deb broke down, apologizing to her daughter that she had to leave. I swallowed hard and prayed I could keep it together.

The video ended and the lights came back up. There were audible sobs from several members of the audience.

"Deb was able to see the video we edited for her daughter on a Friday," I continued. "And she loved it. Two days later, she died." Our only competition is time.

—

There are many questions in my life that I am not able to answer. Why do bad things happen to good people? While we're at it, why do good things happen to bad people? Why does life seem so unfair sometimes?

But one question I never have is "Why did I get cancer?" I never ask that question because I already know the answer: God gave me the ability to tell stories, and cancer gave me the motivation to tell good ones.

I don't look at cancer as a curse, and I don't view it as a blessing, because it is anything but a blessing. Cancer is, however, a perspective changer. In the midst of the chaos, it restored what needed to be the natural order of my being. I learned to embrace life, to search for the meaning in everything, and to fight for those who need someone to fight for them. By bringing me to my knees, it gave me the humility to realize that no matter how much I think I have things figured out, I am not in control.

It sucked having to accept that one.

It also gave me courage, wisdom, and the knowledge that even when cancer takes a body, it does not take the person. Every time

I see a penny on the ground, I say, "Hi, Deb." Our youngest, Benny, prays for Deb every night. Both of my boys also pray for "Framily," which covers just about everyone they know.

    I didn't start out my life's journey wanting to be an activist. I never thought I was strong enough to make a difference. Family, friends, and circumstances proved me wrong. When I look at my life now, I know that everything that has happened—good and bad, happy and sad—has led me to where I am. And for that, I am eternally grateful.

    Even for you, cancer. Bastard.

# EPILOGUE:
## YOUR SERVICES ARE NO LONGER REQUIRED

"**M**ay I help you?"

The student at the Washington University Reproductive Medicine Center looked bored. I couldn't blame him. It was a pretty drab office. Lots of taupe. A ficus tree could have really spruced the place up.

"Yes, I'm not going to renew my membership," I said.

"What do you mean, membership?" It was probably the first time the poor bastard had looked up from his book all morning.

I produced a sheet of paper from my pocket and handed it to him. It was a renewal notice for my bank shot from over a decade prior.

"I'm not going to renew my membership."

I handed the paper to the kid, which he took from me and read. "That's fine, sir."

"Is there anything I need to sign?"

"Are you over eighteen?"

I stared at him. "Really?"

"Over eighteen," he said.

He typed a few words into his computer and pulled up my file.

"Would you mind telling me why you'd like to discard your specimen? Are you unhappy with our services?"

What was this, the cable company? I'm not looking to talk to customer retention, kid.

"I don't need them anymore."

"Wow, okay. Congratulations."

"To tell you the truth, I never used them."

"Really?"

My over-share baffled his young mind. I couldn't quite believe I was having this conversation with someone I didn't know, but he was genuinely curious, and genuine curiosity is a rare thing.

"No."

I stumped him.

"So…" The poor guy had no idea what was going on. "…you don't need them?"

"Yes."

"Wait, what?"

This was too much fun, but I had to let him off the hook. I took out my wallet and pulled out a picture of Sam and Ben playing together. I showed it to him, and I could tell that he wasn't quite sure what he was seeing. Then, slowly, it dawned on him. He looked at me and smiled.

"Excellent work," he said.

## 26: YOUR SERVICES ARE NO LONGER REQUIRED

"Thank you, sir."

I put the picture back in my wallet, and my wallet back in my pocket.

"Well…thanks."

And I turned upon my heel and walked out of the office, grinning until it hurt. I always thought that this moment would be the end of everything, but I was wrong.

It was just the end of the beginning.

# ABOUT THE AUTHOR

Dan Duffy is a husband, dad, and storyteller. As a video producer, Dan has spent over fifteen years telling the stories of extraordinary people. A cancer diagnosis in 2002 forced him into the spotlight he usually reserved for others. Dan realized that his diagnosis was not just a random act of chance, and to treat it as such would potentially waste the opportunity to help people with his new found, if not entirely welcome, experience. Drawing on his expertise in visual and auditory mediums, he has now delved into the literary world, bringing a raw, unapologetic, and hilarious look his own battle with cancer, sanity, and survival, but possibly not in that order. Dan's first book, *The Half Book: He's Taking His Ball and Going Home*, is like nothing you've ever read. As Dan has said, "When the cancer elephant enters the conversation, I don't want people to think they have to apologize. I'd rather they ask, 'What kind?'"